INVESTIGATING DISEASE PATTERNS

The Science of Epidemiology

Contents

Preface   ix

1   Epidemics and Science   1

2   The Beginnings of Epidemiology   23

3   Lung Cancer: New Methods of Studying Disease   51

4   Heart Disease: Untangling the Risk Factors   81

5   Hazards in the Environment: Finding "Safe" Levels   109

6   Medicines that Backfire   139

7   Screening Populations: Costs, Risks, and Benefits   165

8   Health Care Services: What Works?   189

9   The Future of Disease and Epidemiology   206

Further Readings   223

Sources of Illustrations   227

Index   233

INVESTIGATING DISEASE PATTERNS

The Science of Epidemiology

Paul D. Stolley

Tamar Lasky

**SCIENTIFIC
AMERICAN
LIBRARY**

A division of HPHLP
New York

Library of Congress Cataloging-in-Publication Data

Stolley, Paul D.
    Investigating disease patterns : the science of epidemiology
  Paul Stolley and Tamar Lasky.
      p. cm.
  Includes bibliographical references and index.
  ISBN 0-7167-5058-9 (hard cover)
  ISBN 0-7167-6024-X (pbk)
  1. Epidemiology.   I. Lasky, Tamar.   II. Title.
  [DNLM: 1. Epidemiology. 2. Epidemiologic Methods. 3. Disease
Outbreaks.   WA 105 S875i 1995]
  RA651.S75   1995
  614.4—dc20
  DNLM/DLC
  for Library of Congress
                                95-14250
                                CIP

ISSN 1040-3213
© 1995, 1998 by Scientific American Library

Printed in the United States of America

Scientific American Library
A division of HPHLP
New York

Distributed by W. H. Freeman and Company,
41 Madison Avenue, New York, NY 10010
Houndmills, Basingstoke RG21 6XS, England

To those small hands that changed my world:
  Anna, Dorie, and Jon.

                              —PDS

To my husband, Lee, and children,
  Daphne and David.

                      —TL

Preface

The science of epidemiology is the foundation of public health policy and preventive medicine and makes a profound contribution to clinical medicine as well. The clinician is interested in diagnosing and treating disease in the individual patient who comes for help. The epidemiologist is similarly interested in the diagnosis and treatment of disease, but the focus of concern is an entire population rather than individual patients. The clinical physician may ask: What is wrong with this patient? What can be done to treat the patient? The epidemiologist asks similar questions about whole communities: What are the leading causes of death or disability in this population? What can be done to lower the rate of disease?

We ardently hope that our book will convey at least some of the excitement, importance, and challenge of the field of epidemiology, which has been an underappreciated branch of medical science. We think it is a fair assessment of its importance to state that most of what is currently known about both the cause and prevention of human disease is a result of the hard and often difficult work of the many epidemiologists around the world who investigate epidemic disease, sometimes at great personal risk. Their contributions to our understanding of diseases as diverse as infectious diseases, cardiovascular disease, cancer, and occupational and environmentally caused illness make up a large portion of this volume.

Epidemiology is fascinating as well when it turns its eye on the practice of medicine itself, as we explore in the book's final chapters. Some of the field's most intriguing tales describe the investigation of diseases unintentionally caused by physicians' own actions, attempts to treat illness gone awry. Moreover, the practitioners of modern medicine depend on epidemiologists to evaluate the effectiveness of their efforts: Do tests that screen for early disease actually lower death rates? Does a course of treatment truly work in most cases?

In preparing this book we have had the excellent and patient editorial help of Susan Moran, Jonathan Cobb, and Diane Cimino Maass of the Scientific American Library, and have benefitted from the knowledgeable eye of Travis Amos, who located most of the photographs. Anna Stolley helped organize the final sections of the book when her father began to feel overwhelmed by the many remaining details. Tamar Lasky's family tolerated a dining room table covered with galleys and cheered her on, and her husband, Lee, came to the rescue with the obscure and wonderful quotation that opens Chapter 5. Hildred Griffeth deserves our thanks for typing most of the manuscript.

We would particularly like to acknowledge the helpful comments of Carol Rice, Ellen Silbergeld, Steve Havas, Roger Sherwin, Valerie Prenger, James M. Melius, and Berton H. Kaplan. It was a special pleasure to have the comments of Philip Kintner, Grinnell College Professor of History, on Chapter 2.

Paul D. Stolley

Tamar Lasky

June 1995

INVESTIGATING DISEASE PATTERNS

The Science of Epidemiology

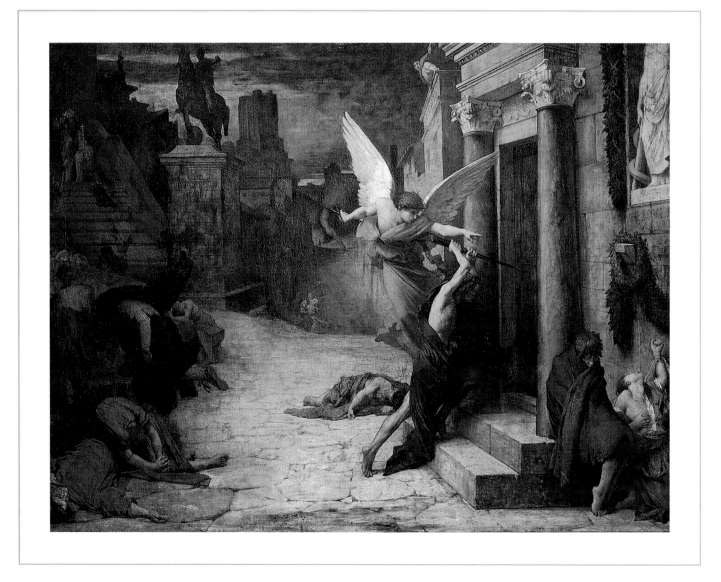

1

Epidemics
and Science

"The mortality in Siena began in May. It was a cruel and horrible thing; and I do not know where to begin to tell of the cruelty and the pitiless ways. It seemed almost everyone became stupefied by seeing the pain. . . . And the victims died almost immediately. They would swell beneath the armpits and in their groins, and fall over while talking. Father abandoned child, wife [abandoned] husband, one brother another; for this illness seemed to strike through breath and sight. And so they died. And none could be found to bury the dead for money or friendship."

This description by Agnola di Tura of the Great Plague of the fourteenth century, also called the Black Death, captures some of the horror of living through a deadly epidemic. Fear and dread disrupt normal social and family relations, and in a severe epidemic, a country's economy and government can be shattered. To appreciate the fear a fatal epidemic disease can inspire, think about how you would feel if you surprised a raccoon in your garage, just after the evening news had reported a surge in rabid wildlife in your county. Now imagine how you might feel if every third person in your community were dying or dead of a strange and inexplicable illness that was sweeping through your city or village. Virtually every inhabitant of Europe faced this terror in the mid-fourteenth century.

The Black Death

TERROR is hardly conducive to investigation, and the plague-beset populations could only speculate wildly about what was happening to them and why. But the scientists of later centuries found the detachment to assess the agony rationally.

The Black Death probably began in Asia in the year 1330, spreading via land and sea trading routes to North Africa, Europe, and the Middle East. The disease is now called bubonic plague, and the bacillus that causes it has the name *Yersina pestis*. The illness caused by this bacillus usually infects the black rat, but several fleas that ordinarily infest these rats will also feed on humans, and if the fleas are infected with the bacillus, they can transmit the infection to humans by their bite (they regurgitate infected material into the bite wound).

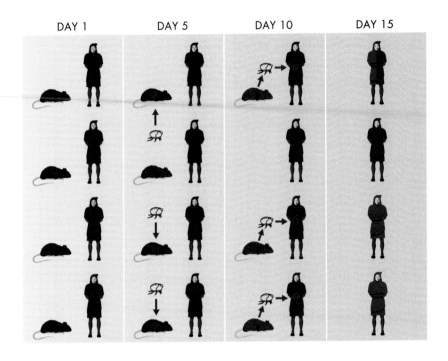

DAY 1   DAY 5   DAY 10   DAY 15

The plague would progress rapidly through a medieval household once a single rat, marked with a large red dot, had been infected. By the fifth day of its infection, the plague-carrying rat would die. The fleas it had harbored would leave its body, carrying the plague to other rats in the house. Once these rats, too, had died, in another five days, the fleas would move on to human hosts. About half the household's human inhabitants would soon die from the plague; a quarter would recover; and another quarter would never become infected.

The complex ecological interrelationship between rat, flea, bacillus, and human must be understood to comprehend the cause and spread of the Black Death during the Middle Ages—and these relationships are still not fully appreciated. There are several theories attempting to explain why the plague epidemic of the fourteenth century was so severe, but none are amenable to proof. The disease may be endemic (that is, more or less constantly present but at a low level) among black rat populations. It is when the rat comes into greater propinquity to humans that its fleas are likely to bite a human host and thus spread the plague bacillus. An animal that spreads a disease is called a *vector* of that disease; the rat flea is the vector of the plague, carrying it from rat to human. Some historians hold that crop failures in China around 1330 caused rats to leave the fields and live in the huts of farmers in an attempt to obtain food; rat fleas were then in closer contact with humans, leading to infection in the human population. The plague can be spread not only by the bite of the infected rat flea, *Xenopsylla cheopis*, but also by the saliva or cough droplets of the infected person. This manner of person-to-person spread is called pneumonic plague. Both routes of infection took place during the Great Plague of the fourteenth century.

The disease is a particularly rapid and horrible one with an incubation period of two to ten days. The first symptoms appear suddenly: high fever, rapid heartbeat, severe headache, and muscular pains. The lymph nodes in the groin, armpits, and neck become swollen and painful and may drain pus. As the disease progresses, hemorrhages appear in the skin; their dark color led the disease to be termed the "black" plague. A severe pneumonia develops, with air hunger and breathing difficulty. Victims cough and gasp for air, the cough spreading the bacilli by droplets to other humans who breathe them in. The death rate among infected persons varies according to the route of infection, dose of bacilli delivered, and the age and condition of the patient; untreated, however, the disease is probably fatal in one-quarter to one-half of those infected.

The effects of this epidemic were devastating. It has been estimated that the population of Europe dropped by 25 to 33 percent during the period from 1330 to 1350—and one must remember that the plague returned several times again over the hundred years following the Great Plague. As the peasants died, agricultural production fell precipitously. Families were dissolved by death or abandonment. Entire villages disappeared. Pogroms were launched against the Jews of Europe, who were thought responsible for the epidemic, even though the Pope pointed out the ludicrousness of this belief.

The depopulation of the countryside led to dramatic political and economic change. The nobility sold off their land: they could no longer find serfs to work it for them. Animal husbandry increased: it was less labor intensive than traditional agriculture. The development of technological advances in industry may have been stimulated by the need to find substitutes for human labor. Yet depopulation also led to the shrinkage of markets for goods, and economic collapse affected parts of Europe following the several plague epidemics.

The Plague Year

Uncontrolled epidemics have stimulated several great literary works, including Boccaccio's *Decameron* (1348–53) and Albert Camus's *The Plague* (1948). Daniel Defoe, the English novelist who wrote *Robinson Crusoe,* later tried his hand at what we now call a "documentary" novel. Writing several decades after the last plague outbreak in London and using historical documentary sources, he recreated the epidemic for his readers in his *Journal of the Plague Year* (1722). Although his statistical accounts of the number of new cases each week and in each parish may bore the modern reader, he is superb when portraying the fear and social disruption generated by a deadly epidemic, as the following passage illustrates.

That there was a great many robberies and wicked practices committed even in this dreadful time I do not deny. The power of avarice was so strong in some that they would run any hazard to steal and to plunder; and particularly in houses where all the families or inhabitants have been dead and carried out, they would break in at all hazards, and without regard to the danger of infection, take even the clothes off the dead bodies and the bed-clothes from others where they lay dead. . . . The inhabitants of the villages adjacent would, in a pity, carry them food, and set it at a distance, that they might fetch it, if they were able; and sometimes they were not able, and the next time they went they should find the poor wretches lie dead and the food untouched. The number of these miserable objects were many, and I know so many that perished thus, and so exactly where, that I believe I could go to the very place and dig their bones up still; for the country people would go and dig a hole at a distance from them, and then with long poles, and hooks at the end of them, drag the bodies into these pits, and then throw the earth in from as far as they could cast it, to cover them, taking notice how the wind blew, and so coming on that side which the seamen call to windward, that the scent of the bodies might blow from them; and thus great numbers went out of the world, who were never known, or any account of them taken, as well within the bills of mortality as without. ●

Optimism and religious concepts were dealt a blow by the terrible mortality from the plague. As one might guess, belief systems to explain it ranged from ascribing the plague to a form of divine retribution for human sins to flat rejection of the concept of a benevolent deity. While a small number sought rational explanations for the plague, probably the majority of the population embraced millennialism and belief in the apocalypse. (After all, not a few religious sages have claimed that the current AIDS epidemic may be a form of divine punishment for proscribed sexual practices.)

What Constitutes an Epidemic?

THE word *epidemic* may lead most people to think of a calamitous occurrence of deadly infectious disease such as the Black Death just described. But medical science defines it as an unusual or increased adverse effect on the health of the population. The word derives from ancient Greek, in which *demos* meant "the people" (as in "democracy"). Endemic disease was "native to" or belonging to the population; epidemic disease was "visiting" or transient. The term *pandemic* ("affecting all the people") now refers to an epidemic that is worldwide in spread.

Today we describe epidemic adverse health effects in terms of time, geography, and the personal characteristics of those who contract the disease or experience the adverse health event. The word epidemic has been used—in our view quite correctly—to describe the 75-year trend in lung cancer, the equally long increase and subsequent decline of coronary artery disease, the several-decade increase in homicide rates in the United States, and the relatively small absolute number of cases of vaginal cancer in adolescent girls due to prenatal exposure to the sex hormone diethylstilbestrol (DES). Suicide can occur in epidemic form, as can acute alcoholism or poisoning from toxic substances in food. Confining the term epidemic to contagious disease presents too narrow a view of the phenomenon. More important, such a restriction might lead to neglect of the powerful tools for investigation available to epidemiologists, the scientists who investigate the causes of modern epidemics.

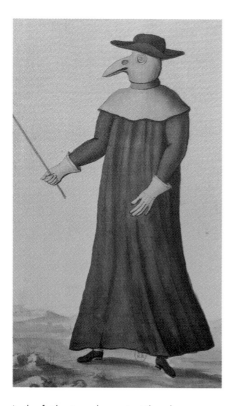

In the futile struggle against the plague, various rituals and costumes were employed by medieval and Renaissance physicians. This costume with the birdlike mask was worn by a physician in Marseilles in the belief that it would protect the wearer from the supposed noxious air presumed to cause plague. The wand contained incense to ward off impurities.

A Modern Epidemic

THE Black Death—with its distinctive symptoms, rapid contagion, and horrific mortality—made its arrival all too clear. But epidemics of new diseases are not always so easily recognized. As the example that follows demonstrates, sometimes the epidemiologist's most significant step in investigating a disease is the realization that it is caused by something wholly new.

A small epidemic of what was originally thought to be juvenile rheumatoid arthritis occurred in and around the town of Lyme, Connecticut, in the mid-1970s. The mother of one of the newly diagnosed young boys heard about several other cases of recently diagnosed arthritis among the children of other town residents. Her curiosity aroused, she asked around to see if there were other cases, spoke to pediatricians and

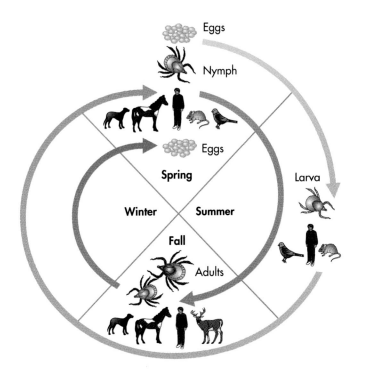

During its two years of life, the tick *I. dammini*—the vector of Lyme disease—feeds three times: once as a larva on the blood of mice or other small mammals; once as a slightly larger nymph on the blood of mice or larger mammals; and once or more as an adult, often on the white-tailed deer. The larva picks up the disease-causing *B. burgdorferi* bacterium from infected mice; most often Lyme disease is transmitted to humans from the bite of an infected nymph.

parents, and began to record her collected data systematically. Along with the mother of another victim, she acted as an epidemiologist. They located on a map the residence of each of the six cases that they had discovered and were surprised to see they were all at the edge of a woods along the Connecticut River. Might the so-called juvenile rheumatoid arthritis actually be a different disorder, somehow related to the location near the woods? The boys did not play together, so person-to-person transmission of some infectious agent was unlikely.

The two women presented their data to the State Health Department and the Rheumatology Division of the Yale University Medical School. Dr. Allen Steere of Yale, a rheumatologist who had previously trained in epidemiology while serving in the Centers for Disease Control (CDC) of the United States Public Health Service, soon recognized that the astute mothers were showing him a disease "cluster." Juvenile rheumatoid arthritis is a rare disease that occurs sporadically, but this arthritis was mysteriously clustered in boys living near one another; moreover, the onsets of the disease were within a few months — a cluster in time as well as in space. Dr. Steere knew of somewhat similar diseases that were transmitted by the bite of ticks or fleas. Since some of the parents of the young cases reported a tick bite and rash a few weeks before the onset of the arthritis, he hypothesized that the cluster of arthritis cases might have arisen from an infection transmitted to humans by ticks that usually parasitize woodland animals.

Eventually the cause of the arthritis and the mode of transmission were elucidated. In fact, a new disease had been discovered. The cause of what is now called Lyme disease (after the town of Lyme) is a spiral-shaped bacterium identified by Willy Burgdorfer and named after him: *Borrelia burgdorferi*. The tiny tick that transmits this pathogenic microbe is named *Ixodes dammini*, and it is found in woods and grassy areas. Unfortunately, its range has expanded so widely that this local outbreak proved to be the harbinger of a significant new threat to public health in many areas.

In setting forth the symptoms and other characteristics of Lyme disease, Dr. Steere and his associates were carrying out one of the epidemiologist's primary activities: the description and classification of diseases.

The microorganism that causes Lyme disease, called *Borrelia burgdorferi*, is a spiral-shaped bacterium of the type known as a spirochete.

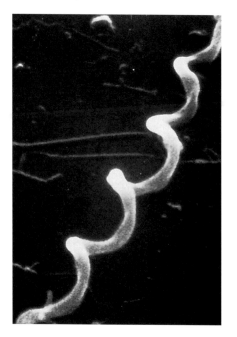

The Natural History of Disease

Natural history — a term that may bring to mind painstaking observations of the natural world conducted by Darwin, Audubon, or Fabre — remains appropriate in describing an aspect of disease crucial from the epidemiologist's perspective. Just as nineteenth-century scientists depended on field observation as their principal source of data, elevating amateur naturalists' jottings into disciplined and meticulous records, so epidemiology must take the ordinary course of a disease and the established causal factors into account if explanations are to be found for an epidemic increase in the disease's spread, virulence, or typical victim profile. A devastating example is that of the polio virus, which before the present century was endemic throughout the world; almost everyone was infected, but paralytic disease was less common. Only after modern sanitation had preserved a substantial population in the United States and Scandinavia from infection as infants (polio is spread in contaminated water supplies or person-to-person by the fecal-oral route) was the natural course of the virus altered: lacking immunity, schoolchildren and adults encountering infection for the first time suffered paralytic illness. ●

A full description of a disease covers many facets. What is the spectrum of the disease from its mildest form to its most severe? What is the "natural history" of the disease (its ordinary course)? If left untreated, will it resolve or progress?

What, moreover, are the best ways to group diseases? The answers that best serve epidemiology and public health may differ from those of ordinary medical practice. Lung cancer, emphysema, chronic bronchitis, and coronary heart disease might be grouped as "cigarette-induced diseases" for example — sometimes a more useful classification than dividing these disorders on the basis of the affected organ system.

The outbreak of Lyme disease described above has in common with other epidemics that its victims had encountered some factor — in this case, the spirochete *Borrelia burgdorferi*. Epidemiologists view their work as the search for a relationship between two factors. One, called the exposure, refers to any factor that can affect a person's health. The second is the disease itself. Just as "disease" can refer to any adverse health condition, from an illness to an injury to an addiction, so too an exposure need not be a germ or a toxin; it can be a habit (like smoking), a behavior (like driving while intoxicated), or a defective gene (as in cystic fibrosis).

The task of the epidemiologist is to find a relationship between a factor and a disease and to decide if that observed relationship is causal: Did the exposure in fact result in the disease? Whether an epidemiologist can track down the cause of an epidemic depends to a great extent on how well he or she has characterized that epidemic. The real genius of epidemiology is that it characterizes an outbreak of a disease not just by description of symptoms but by finding out in great detail who gets the disease, for the characteristics of the victims often suggest a probable cause.

How Are Epidemics Characterized?

LIKE a detective, the epidemiologist pursues the most promising clues—and the population affected is the usual starting point for the epidemiologist faced with a mysterious epidemic. Who is getting sick? Are they the young? the old? males? females? persons with certain occupations? The discovery of so-called Legionnaire's disease illustrates the value of characterizing the affected population as completely as possible. The victims of this unusual and often fatal lobar pneumonia were primarily middle-aged or aged men who were members of the American Legion. All had attended the American Legion Annual Convention in Philadelphia in 1976 and had either stayed in or attended meetings at a particular hotel, the Bellevue-Stratford. To explain this disease, one had to explain why few women were affected, why family members of the victims were spared—and account, moreover, for the fact that most of those ill had patronized a particular hotel. Once all the facts were gathered, the search for a cause focused on the hotel. It turned out that the transmissable agent that causes Legionnaire's disease had multiplied in reservoirs of heated water that formed part of the Bellevue-Stratford's air-conditioning system. This agent, a bacterium, was then distributed throughout the hotel in the circulated air.

Certain diseases display unusual distribution patterns by gender, and this may eventually be useful in helping to uncover their causes. For example, systemic lupus erythematosus (SLE), a collagen-vascular disease that can produce skin, joint, and kidney damage, is found eight times more commonly in females than in males, for reasons still unclear. Diseases often thought to be exclusive to women are sometimes found in men—breast cancer is about a hundred times less common in men than women in the United States, but it does occur occasionally in males. The study of the risk factors in men, where it is so rare, may be revealing (the same is true of SLE). The reasoning is that when a disease does occur in a normally resistant "host" or population, it may be due to overwhelming presence of the causal agent(s) or risk factors, which may then be more easily identified.

Some cancers tend to occur in men because males are more often exposed to what Dr. Alice Hamilton, the first American occupational medical practitioner, called the "dangerous trades." Thus angiosarcoma of the liver in those working with vinyl chloride, and lung cancer in chemical workers exposed to bis-chlor methyl ether (BCME), occurred in young men, which helped to confirm the occupational etiology of these tumors.

However, an epidemic of occupational cancer did occur in females some decades ago in the 1920s and 1930s. Workers, mainly young women, were employed to apply radioactive substances to watch faces and dials, making them luminous in the dark. Each would "point" her paintbrush by putting the brush tip in her mouth and so ingested this radioactive paint. Since the paint had a long radioactive life, it continued to emit radiation when it was absorbed into the body and stored in the lymphatic system, jawbone, and liver. This radiation produced some cancers in these occupationally exposed women, especially in the jaw.

In addition to age and gender, geography helps to characterize an epidemic. Placing cases of an epidemic onto a map is called "spot-mapping," and the technique can be revealing. After the successful mass polio immunization campaigns of the late 1950s and early 1960s in the

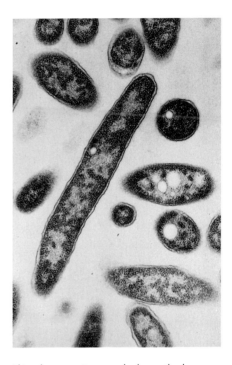

This electron micrograph shows the bacterium that causes Legionnaires' disease, *Legionella pneumophila*. One of the authors (Paul Stolley) investigated an outbreak of this disease at a Washington, D.C., hospital in 1966, ten years before the causative agent was identified. Frozen sera from the victims was tested a decade later and proved that this bacterium was the agent of infection.

Mining has long been recognized as a source of occupational illnesses. Uranium miners, for example, run the risk of developing lung cancer from the radioactive dust they inhale while they work. This Navajo miner had cancer of the lung at the time this photograph was taken.

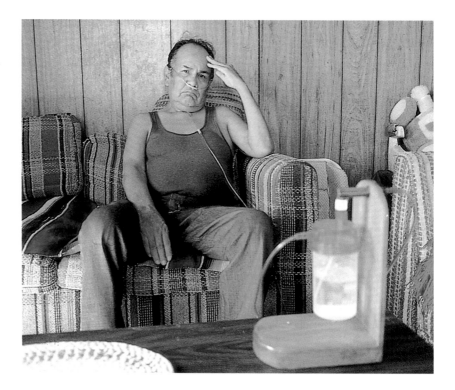

United States, most new cases of wild or naturally occurring polio popped up along the border with Mexico in recent immigrants who had not received the vaccine.

Sometimes cancers distribute geographically in peculiar patterns that seem to provide a strong clue about the cause of the particular cancer. Esophageal cancer, for example, is very common around the Caspian littoral, but the reasons are not clear, although chemicals in soil and certain eating habits have been suggested, particularly the drinking of a commonly used beverage at extraordinarily hot temperatures.

At times, characterizing an epidemic by the religion or ethnicity of the area in which it occurs can be informative. A small number of cases of human infestation with the large fish tapeworm in New York City occurred almost exclusively in Jewish housewives. It was traced to the ingestion of raw fish while making gefilte fish for the Passover meal. The housewife would taste it before cooking to check on the seasoning. Unfortunately, the whitefish came from Canadian lakes where the tapeworm was present and infecting the fish.

In the United States, the information in birth and death records or about specific diseases like cancer is often collected with "race" indicated on the form. Social, educational, and economic status is much less often collected routinely. Since African Americans tend to have lower incomes and educational attainment than the Caucasian population, as a result of systematic and long-term discrimination, the health status of these citizens can be affected. Thus "race" sometimes serves as a proxy or surrogate measure for poverty and lower socioeconomic class. The biological and genetic interpretation of health differences must be approached very cautiously, since the environmental and social conditions of those persons classified under "race" may be the most important determinant of their health status.

Since few people have a homogeneous racial or ethnic background, the concept of "race" may be an outmoded and anachronistic formulation. The high infant mortality rate found in African Americans has led to the hypothesis that inadequate and delayed prenatal care (rather than any genetic reason) is the probable cause of the twofold difference in these rates when African Americans are compared to Caucasian Americans. In spite of these caveats and difficulties in interpretation, classifying epidemics by the "racial" composition of the population affected has provided useful clues about the cause and mode of spread of disease. For example, the cancer malignant melanoma is very rare in African Americans and much more common among blue-eyed and fair-skinned Caucasians. This has lent some support to the hypothesis that this tumor is caused by sun injury to unprotected skin.

Genetic susceptibility is sometimes a vital consideration, as we know from sickle-cell disease (in African Americans) and Tay-Sachs disease (found in Ashkenazi Jews). But medical investigators have been misled in the past about the relationship of ethnicity and disease frequency because they failed to take into account the population from which the initial cases were derived. When thromboangiitis obliterans (Buerger's disease) was first described by Buerger in the 1920s, he stated that it had a predilection for persons of Jewish European ancestry. This disease of the peripheral arterial system (found almost exclusively in heavy cigarette smokers) has since been shown to occur all over the world, but Buerger worked at a hospital (Mount Sinai in Manhattan) where most of the patients at that time had European Jewish ancestry. This simple error, once embedded in the medical literature, has been hard to remove in subsequent years, though later studies provide little evidence that a particular ethnicity or religion places an individual at greater risk of getting the disorder.

As the examples above show, the epidemiologist must characterize the affected population shrewdly, sizing it up without being led astray by red herrings or irrelevant detail. The careful marshalling and evaluation of facts are the keys to the successful field investigation of epidemics, as the following example illustrates:

Field Work: Investigating an Epidemic

DURING the summer of 1964 a peculiar illness was reported from the tri-city area of the state of Washington near the Hanford atomic bomb production facility. This area of Washington has a semi-arid, desertlike climate with scant rainfall. In addition to the bomb production facility, the main economic activity is dairy farming and agriculture dependent upon irrigation water derived from the tributaries to Columbia River.

All of the cases initially reported, ten in total, were teenage boys who complained of headache, fever, and malaise. All seemed to recover, and most had been treated with antibiotics even though the most frequent diagnosis with which they were labeled was "atypical meningitis" (which, in 1964, was presumed to be of viral etiology and thus not treatable with antibiotics). A team of epidemiologists from the Epidemic Intelligence Service of the federal Centers for Disease Control was dispatched to aid the state and county health authorities in their investigation.

The team first decided to look for additional cases of the disease that might not have been recognized or reported. They searched through hospital admission logs for disease categories that fit the same clinical pic-

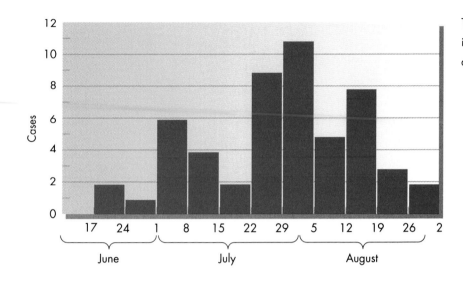

The Hanford area epidemic took place in three waves throughout the summer of 1964.

ture as the one the teenage boys had exhibited. They conducted a telephone survey of physicians in the area and asked them if they had seen similar patients, and they arranged for the local newspaper to run articles about the disease. They requested that the parents of possibly affected persons or the persons themselves call in and discuss their illness with the staff. Eventually, they located 61 persons that fit their case-definition of this unknown disease: a clinical picture of headache, joint aches, fever, and an abnormal urinalysis.

When the attack rate was graphed (number of cases plotted against time), the graph produced showed that the epidemic began June 20, 1964, and ended August 30, 1964. The cases were tabulated according to age and sex. All the cases occurred in teenagers. Of the 61 cases, 53 were male and only 8 female.

The epidemiologists developed a working hypothesis to help organize the epidemic investigation after serological tests revealed that most of the affected teenagers had antibodies to *Leptospira* microorganisms, suggesting a recent infection by this bacterium. The epidemiologic concept of causality goes beyond identification of the pathogenic or chemical agents of disease to consider routes of transmission and exposure, as well as individual susceptibility to illness. What was the vector of this particular outbreak?

Distribution of Cases by Age and Sex

Age	Male	Female	Total
Under 12	0	0	0
12	2	0	2
13	2	1	3
14	6	0	6
15	7	1	8
16	12	2	14
17	16	0	16
18	3	0	3
19	0	1	1
Over 19	0	0	0
Totals	48	5	53

A species of *Leptospira,* the spirochete that caused the epidemic among children in the Hanford area. The spirochete had gotten into the irrigation canal water when infected cattle, wading in the water to keep cool during the hot summer months, urinated into the canal.

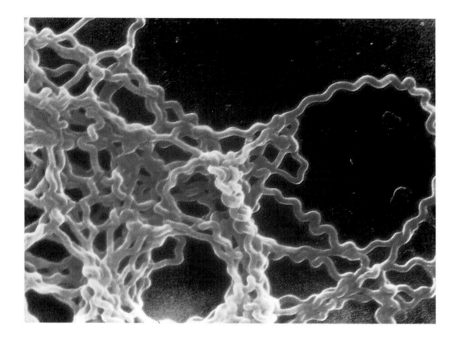

Knowing that the disease leptospirosis is spread by direct contact with the organism, which is excreted in the urine of affected rodents and large animals such as cattle, the team postulated that the "vehicle" for the infection was probably contaminated water. They developed a questionnaire to administer to the cases and also to a group of unaffected teenagers who attended the same schools. The questionnaire was short and simple, often an advisable strategy when trying to collect information from volunteers, and focused on symptoms of illness during the summer and places where the schoolchildren may have gone swimming. This interest in swimming holes was prompted by many of the earliest identified cases giving a history of having gone swimming in the same place—an irrigation channel where the water came bubbling up from a pumping station to enter a concrete-lined canal that was wide and had a ledge from which to jump into the maelstrom.

The results of the questionnaire are shown in the table on the facing page. One can see that most of the cases had been to the irrigation canal swimming hole, called "the Bubbles" by the children, whereas few of the

Response to Questions

	Swam			Did not swim			Difference in attack rates
	Total	Sick	Attack rate	Total	Sick	Attack rate	
The "Bubbles"	594	126	21.2%	5,164	248	4.8%	16.4%
Irrigation water (not the "Bubbles")	1,123	136	12.1%	4,041	112	2.8%	9.3%

healthy children had used this swimming hole. Veterinarians joined the investigative team, and an aerial survey of the irrigation canals established that a herd of cattle were kept upstream near the canal. These cattle were often seen immersed in the canal to cool off during the heat of the summer, and of course would urinate into the water. The veterinarians took blood samples and collected urine from a sample of the herd closest to the "Bubbles." The cows had antibodies to *Leptospira pomona,* and the

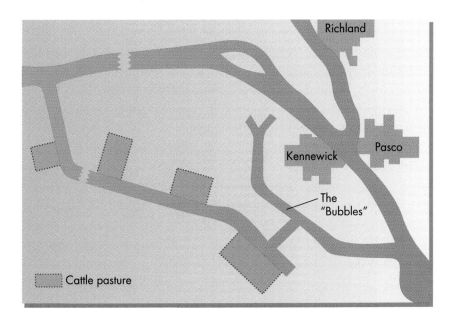

The infected cattle grazed in unfenced pastures adjacent to the irrigation canal and so could easily enter the canal and contaminate the water. The *Leptospira* probably invaded the human host through the conjunctive membrane of the eye or through scratches in the skin.

organism was cultured from the urine of some of the cattle, indicating a recent infection of the herd. The affected teenagers with the "strange disease" were tested for antibodies to this particular strain of *Leptospira,* and most showed antibodies. Those children who had not been swimming in irrigation water had no antibodies to *Leptospira.* The mystery of the epidemic was solved.

Epidemiology and the Scientific Method

IN each of the epidemics cited in this chapter, the characteristic sex or locale or recreational site of the victims was a clue that helped investigators develop a reasonable hypothesis about the exposure that led to the disease. A hypothesis—idea or conjecture about the relationship between events—underlies the epidemiologist's actions and inquiries. In common with other scientific fields, epidemiology begins with formal statements of hypotheses: conceptual statements that describe the expected relationship between events and that are subject to statistical testing.

The scientific method depends on the capacity to put forth new ideas, combined with a willingness to subject each idea to the tests of reality, followed by an ability to incorporate the information derived from tests. Whether the tests (experimental or observational) allow one to reject or accept the null hypothesis, the testing process provides useful data that can be used to revise the hypothesis or to develop new hypotheses.

The philosopher of science Sir Karl Popper expressed many of these ideas and has greatly influenced the epidemiologic approach to hypotheses. He coined the term "falsification" to express the concept that scientific theories are not proven by repetition of results but rather survive because they successfully withstand refutation (falsification). His example of the black swan makes this point quite clearly. Suppose you have a hypothesis that *all swans are white.* You observe, say, ten thousand swans, and they are all white. Another scientist repeats your efforts and observes another ten thousand swans: they, too, are all white. So far the theory is standing up well. The repetition helped to strengthen it—but if only a *single* black swan is sighted, this falsifies the theory: it is no longer tenable. Popper asserted that scientific statements have to be formulated in a manner that subjects them to the possibility of falsification. One of the important demarcating criteria between science and nonscience, according to Popper, is this formulation of statements in a manner permitting falsification.

The formation of an epidemiological hypothesis involves a synthesis of general biological, health, and social science theory, as well as observations of cases, case series, or data trends in different areas over time. Many epidemiologic investigations and discoveries were initiated because an astute clinician observed a few cases of a disease, then formulated a hypothesis about the cause of the condition. Some examples are the associations between rubella exposure during pregnancy and congenital cataracts of the eye, occupational lead exposure and kidney damage, and cigarette smoking and lung cancer.

Working with live human populations imposes special constraints that scientists with animal disease models or laboratory bacterial cultures need not consider. Ethical concerns rule out many experiments that would offer epidemiologists clear and unequivocal answers. To meet this special challenge, they have instead evolved several kinds of specialized research strategies, principally the case-control (retrospective) method and the cohort (prospective) study.

In the case-control study the investigator starts by assembling a group of persons with the disease of interest and then inquires into those items in their past (retrospective) history that may provide a clue to the cause of the illness. These persons are compared to a control group of otherwise similar individuals who are either healthy or may have diseases other than the one under investigation. Something like this technique was used by the team in Washington state. Another example was the investigation of "toxic shock," a disorder overwhelmingly affecting women, where the case-control method quickly pinpointed the most common exposure among the cases: use of a new, highly absorbent tampon.

In the cohort study the epidemiologist assembles a group of people with a common exposure (working in an asbestos factory, for example),

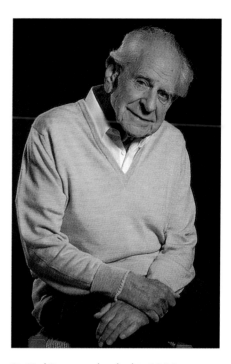

Sir Karl Popper, who died in 1994 at over 90 years of age, was the most widely known philosopher of science during the past half century. His idea that the falsification of hypotheses is a key feature of the scientific method has gained great currency and helped guide the research programs of a number of epidemiologists and other scientists.

and then follows their medical destiny. Do workers exposed to asbestos have higher rates of lung cancer and cancer of the mesothelium (lining of the pleural cavity) than a comparison group of workers not exposed to asbestos? Do the cigarette smokers among them have a higher incidence of lung cancer and emphysema than the nonsmokers? Careful records assembled over years or decades allow the researchers to assess the significance of the exposure in the unfolding health histories of the chosen cohort by contrast with their unexposed counterparts.

The scientific method is central to scientific exploration, development of knowledge, and the testing of claims. Epidemiology is the scientific building block of the fields of public health and preventive medicine. In times of severe health crisis it brings reason to bear on epidemic human suffering and death, combating not only the contemporary equivalents of the Black Death but the panic, superstition, and social disruption that threaten to accompany them. On a daily basis, it represents the application of the scientific method to questions involving the everyday physical well-being of populations. The uses of epidemiology include not only searching for causes of disease (as we have seen in this chapter) but also evaluating the workings of health services, as will be discussed in Chapter 8. Epidemiology provides the tools by which medical scientists follow the rise and fall of disease: Which diseases are increasing over time and which are decreasing? To get a true picture of disease, knowlege of its distribution across the full spectrum of a population is often needed, since studying those cases that come to attention as hospital admissions can bias the observations to the most severe and refractory cases, which may also be the most advanced. The "hidden" cases of illness are often pictured graphically using the image of an "iceberg" of disease—only the tip of the iceberg is visible in the large teaching hospital, while the remainder of less severe or early cases lies hidden "underwater" in the community.

Epidemiologists have made important contributions to the understanding of specific diseases such as cancer, cardiovascular disease, occupational illnesses, and those diseases (called iatrogenic) caused inadvertently by physicians in their efforts to diagnose and treat. These specialized areas of epidemiology each have a chapter devoted to them.

Changing ecological conditions affect human disease by altering the relation of humankind with parasites and the microbial world and by introducing new threats to human health into the environment as a consequence of industrial processes, use of pesticides, and other human activities and technologies. Epidemiology helps us to recognize these threats and control them, as well as providing an "early warning" surveillance system. Our final chapter deals with some of these issues and tries to predict what the major threats to human health will be and what challenges epidemiology will face as we enter the third millennium.

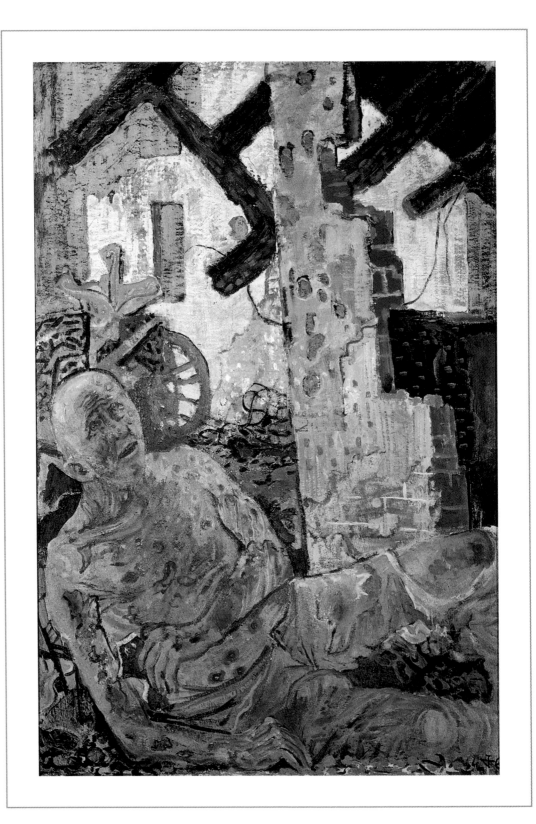

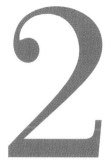

The Beginnings of Epidemiology

PEOPLE HAVE always wondered about illness, its
sources, and its meaning in their lives. This painting by Otto Dix—translating the biblical story of
Job to the ruins of postwar Europe—suggests
the connections between poverty, urban environments, war, and disease found by some of the
earliest epidemiologists.

"The wrath of God," as the well-known epidemiologist Charles-Edward Amory Winslow reminded us in 1943, was no doubt the oldest theory of disease causation; he quoted from Exodus (9:14): "For now I will stretch out mine hand, that I may smite thee and thy people with pestilence." A similar vision shapes the first book of the Iliad, and belief in disease as divine punishment survives to the present day. But Hippocrates (460–377 B.C.), in the *Epidemics*, meticulously described the symptoms and course of different illnesses, relating these to the seasons, geographical area, and types of people associated with each. By recording observations and suggesting nonsupernatural causal hypotheses, he founded the rational approach to the understanding of disease.

The roots of modern medicine and epidemiology, however, are to be recognized in the seventeenth century. Thomas Sydenham, a physician of that century called "the English Hippocrates," was often cited by texts of the early twentieth century as the "father of epidemiology." His careful descriptions of dysentery, gout, malaria, measles, smallpox, syphilis, and tuberculosis were essential in the definition of these diseases as distinct entities and, eventually, in establishing the germ theory of disease. Sydenham wrote, "All diseases then ought to be reduced to certain and determinate kinds, with the same exactness as we see it done by botanic writers in their treatises of plants." He reasoned that biological uniqueness could be attributed to specific diseases—a fact that had to wait two hundred years to be confirmed by the discoveries of microbiologists.

Epidemiology texts of the last thirty years no longer mention Sydenham's achievement; epidemiology and medicine have progressed so far that it may be difficult to see the connection between Sydenham's work in describing diseases and present-day epidemiologic issues. But recognition and description of a disease are the first steps in understanding and ultimately preventing it, and they remain crucial in epidemiology, as the doctors who recognized the disease AIDS demonstrated in the early 1980s.

Thomas Sydenham (1624–1689), the "English Hippocrates."

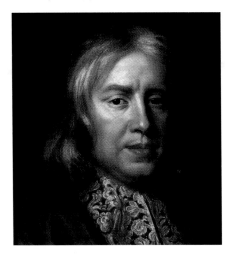

The Seventeenth Century: Describing Disease and Counting Events

TWO British contemporaries of Sydenham advanced another dimension of epidemiologic endeavor: the counting of disease events. Sir William Petty and John Graunt worked together using numerical data to describe patterns of mortality. Of the two, William Petty was the more colorful personality. The son of a clothier and dyer, Petty went to sea at the age of fourteen, studied mathematics and navigation in France, served with the British Navy, then returned to the Continent to study medicine. By 1650 he was deputy to the professor of anatomy at Brasenose College, Oxford, and had been appointed professor of music at Gresham College, London. This last appointment, apparently received through the intervention of the Graunt family, marked the beginning of the friendship between Graunt and Petty. Petty went on to become Surveyor General of Ireland in 1652, published the first map of Ireland, received a knighthood (1662), and, in the same year, joined with eleven other men to found The Royal Society. He published 160 works on such diverse subjects as cartography, economics, mortality, population growth, and navigation. He proposed the establishment of a central government agency to collect data on births, marriages, burials, houses, ages, sex, occupations, revenue, education, and trade—an idea not implemented in Great Britain until the nineteenth century.

Petty also envisioned the uses of such data; he suggested the construction of tables by age and mortality, thus anticipating the later development of actuarial tables to compare mortality and life expectancy in different populations. Petty framed questions to be answered by the data.

> Whether they [viz. fellows and licentiates of the College of Physicians] take as much medicine and remedies as the like number of any other society.

Whether of 1,000 patients to the best physicians, aged of any decade, there do not die as many as out of the inhabitants of places where there dwell no physicians.

Whether of 100 sick of acute diseases who use physicians, as many die and in misery, as where no art is used, or only chance.

His mind grasped the full range of epidemiological thinking: the posing of questions in the form of testable hypotheses, the collection of data to support or refute hypotheses, and the development of statistical tools to summarize numerical data. This far-thinking man had his hand in many other activities (such as the development of a double-bottom ship) and his pockets well lined: in 1685 he estimated his

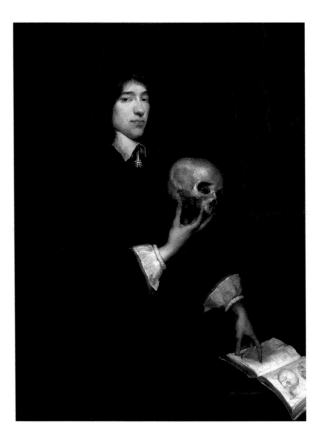

Sir William Petty (1623–1687)—a man of many interests and accomplishments.

personal worth at 45,000 pounds. After his death, his widow was raised to the peerage, and the title passed through his daughter to the marquises of Lansdowne. Although Petty did not live to see his family honored, its elevation in status seems to have been a fulfillment of his ambitions, which he expressed in a rhyme that he composed for his daughter: "My pretty little Pussling and my daughter Ann; That shall be a countesse, if her poppa can." Petty was a wonderful mixture of talent and ambition successfully realized.

By contrast, there is little to say about John Graunt, a long-time acquaintance of Petty's. The son of an influential tradesman in the City of London, he became a haberdasher and, through his activity in civic affairs, a councilman. His one published work, *Observations on the Bills of Mortality*, earned him admission to The Royal Society in 1663 and secured his place in the history of epidemiology. In *Observations*, Graunt analyzed parish records of christenings, burials, and causes of death; without knowing the ages of the dead, he drew inferences about life expectancy and patterns of disease. For example, he concluded that 36 percent of live births died before the age of six. He observed that more males are born than females, a factor balanced by higher male mortality from violence, war, and other causes. Graunt became bankrupt after London's Great Fire of 1666, dropped out of The Royal Society, and died in 1674.

Some contemporaries of Petty and Graunt (including the astronomer Edmund Halley, also of The Royal Society) attributed the *Observations* to Petty, a dispute over authorship that has been occasionally revived to the present day. This unresolved debate signifies that there were at least two men (Graunt and Petty) known to have an interest in the numerical analysis of mortality records. The two men were friends and collaborators, however, and their work was received with interest, suggesting an active and receptive intellectual climate. The work of Graunt and Petty did not make an immediate contribution to the understanding of disease, but it helped establish an interest in the collection and organization of information that would allow epidemiologic methods to develop in the centuries to follow.

A drawing of anthrax bacilli by Robert
Koch, who discovered these rod-shaped,
pathogenic microogranisms in 1876.

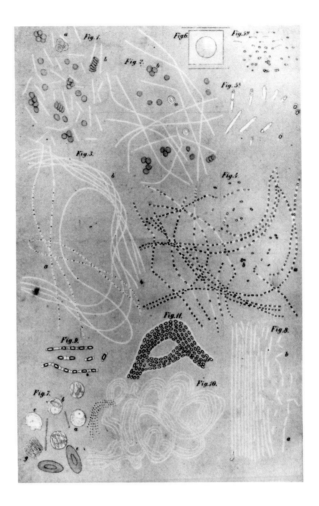

The Century of Statistics and Microbiology

DURING the nineteenth century, as comprehension of disease advanced,
the intellectual community embraced the use of statistics to frame and
answer questions on a variety of issues. Victorian zeal for social reform
together with the era's scientific progress created a fertile climate for the
development of epidemiologic techniques used on all levels: for describ-

ing diseases, identifying their causes, developing records to keep track of disease, and preventing diseases.

As predicted by Sydenham, microbiologists succeeded in identifying specific living organisms with individual, clinically defined diseases. The work of Louis Pasteur, Robert Koch, and others provided biological understanding of the infectious disease process by isolating pathogens associated with particular diseases and demonstrating the infectious properties of the different pathogens.

Pasteur, the founder of modern microbiology, intuitively understood the principles of epidemiology. Not only did his work help to clarify the germ theory of disease, but he went beyond to point out behavioral practices that influenced the transmission of illness and, further, to describe host factors that affected susceptibility. He demonstrated that the burial of anthrax-infected sheep in fields where healthy sheep were pastured led to transmission of anthrax to the grazing sheep. The bacteria survived in the soil and were transmitted to the sheep when sharp stalks of mown grass or stubble cut their legs. Pasteur thus proposed two practical ways to reduce the incidence of anthrax by interfering with transmission: he encouraged farmers to bury anthrax-killed sheep in fields not used for grazing, and he suggested that sheep graze where there was no stubble. Pasteur, recognizing the pathogenic cause of disease, simultaneously understood the causal relationship between farming practices and animal mortality. When Pasteur expanded his research to host factors, he was able to demonstrate how one can alter an animal's susceptibility to disease. He took hens that were normally resistant to anthrax and lowered their body temperatures. After their body temperature had been lowered by cold baths, the hens died if they were inoculated with anthrax bacilli. Hens immersed in cold water, but not inoculated with anthrax, did not die. He demonstrated that bacterial disease depends on the presence of a pathogen as well as host susceptibility to the pathogen.

Application of knowledge about the bacterial cause of many diseases demonstrated other possibilities of reducing illness and mortality. The work of Sir Joseph Lister in preventing infections during surgery is an example. In 1865 Lister became aware of Pasteur's work demonstrating that the air contains invisible particles that can produce fermentation or decomposition. By 1866 Lister had applied this concept to a specific problem, the infection of wounds after surgery, and was experimenting with applying carbolic acid and other antiseptics to wounds. His success in putting this new "germ theory" of disease to use to prevent infection provided further confirming evidence for the theory.

William Farr: A Victorian Data Collector

AGAINST the backdrop of a developing theory of disease origins and advances in microbiology, biology, and medicine, the growing field of statistics was also being harnessed to the study of disease. Victorians were in-

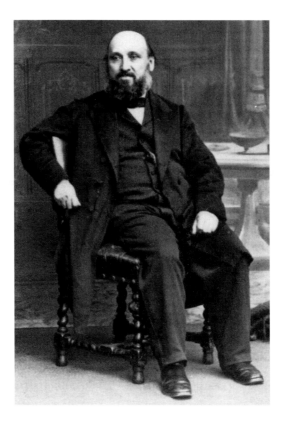

William Farr (1807–1883), who for more than forty years supervised the growth of England's system of vital statistics.

fatuated with statistics. Numerous statistical societies were founded throughout England in the 1830s and 1840s, including the London Statistical Society in 1834. Statistics were collected and applied to problems of economics, prison reform, education, sanitation, and the general reform of society. In 1838 William Petty's vision of a centralized data collection agency was realized with the establishment of the General Register Office to record all births and deaths. By good fortune, the right man was available to run the new agency. William Farr, appointed in 1839 as compiler of statistical abstracts and later as superintendent, served until 1880. During his long tenure at the General Register Office, he collaborated with other influential thinkers of the day (John Snow, Florence Nightingale, and others) and developed the epidemiologic uses of vital statistics and other centralized data sources.

Farr, similar to Petty in being something of a self-made man, was the son of a farm laborer. The farmer to whom Farr was apprenticed at age eight became his patron, encouraging him in school and leaving him an inheritance that enabled Farr to study medicine and statistics in Paris. There he studied under Pierre Louis, the renowned French physician and developer of the "numerical method" in medicine. Upon his return to England, Farr began writing articles for *The Lancet* and became an editor of that journal in 1835. In 1839 he wrote a history of medicine as a social institution, clearly distinguishing his subject from the history of the facts and principles of medicine. "The state of Medical Science is only one of the elements of the inquiry; for the problem is—given a certain quantity of science, how has that science been brought into contact with the people, by what class of persons, by what institutions, and with what effect." How well this statement, an outlook incorporated into the realm of epidemiology more than 100 years later, expresses the public health, community medicine orientation of the twentieth century.

In his work at the General Register Office, Farr developed techniques for data collection, categorized occupations and diseases, published reports, generated questions for further study, and collaborated with other intellectuals. Farr was involved in the first modern census in Great Britain (1841), where for the first time written questionnaires were filled out all over England on the same night. One of Farr's innovations was his categorization of occupations into five classes and eighteen orders (no doubt recalling the use of these terms in taxonomic classification of animals and plants); employing the census data, Farr grouped people by age and occupation. Farr also, beginning in 1839, developed a system for classifying diseases; it underwent several revisions, and the third one, adopted in 1860, was used for another twenty years. Again adopting taxonomic terms (classes and orders), Farr grouped health disorders into five classes: zymotic, constitutional, local, developmental, and violent. The "zymotic" class included epidemic, endemic, and contagious illnesses (*zymotic* is an archaic word for infectious disease). The second class, "constitutional," included gout, dropsy, cancer, and tubercular diseases. "Local" diseases comprised problems of eight organ systems; "developmental" diseases included those of childhood, old age, women, and faulty nutrition. To the fifth class, "violent," were assigned accidents, battle deaths, homicides, suicides, and executions.

Classification systems rarely satisfy everyone, and both praise and criticism were heaped on Farr. The debate reflected scientific and administrative questions of the day and issues still relevant: How should a system of disease categories relate to the causes and the appearances of given diseases? How do these diseases relate to causes of death, and how can physicians use such a system in a consistent and informative way when filling out death certificates?

John Snow and the London Cholera Epidemics

FARR fostered the development of the statistical approach to understanding and preventing disease in his collaborations with John Snow and Florence Nightingale. John Snow is well known for advancing the use of anesthesia (he administered chloroform to Queen Victoria during the birth of Prince Leopold) and, while conducting an active practice, also undertook a famous investigation of the British cholera epidemics of 1849 and 1853. Cholera had ravaged India in 1818, and descriptions of the terrible disease reached England along with news of cholera's spread to the Middle East, Russia, the Balkans, and Germany. In 1831 the first British

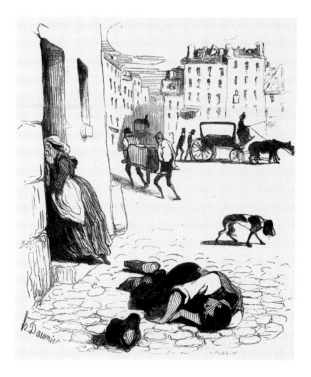

Honoré Daumier's wood engraving of a street in cholera-stricken Paris, rendered in 1840. Cholera struck its victims and killed them within two to three days.

case of cholera was diagnosed in the port city of Sunderland. The patient died after three days of vomiting and diarrhea, and other cases followed, leading to the epidemic of 1832 and the deaths of five to seven thousand persons. When a second cholera epidemic occurred in England in 1848–9, the medical community responded by forming the London Epidemiological Society, of which John Snow was an active participant.

Snow's investigations correctly concluded that the disease was transmitted through contaminated drinking water. He wrote up a clear description of his activities and his thought process in *On the Mode of Communication of Cholera*, published in 1854. Snow's reasoning began with the observation that the spread of cholera appeared to follow international travel routes. Consecutive cases suggested some mode of transmission: they were more numerous than one would expect by mere coincidence. Assuming that some diseases are communicable, Snow cited syphilis

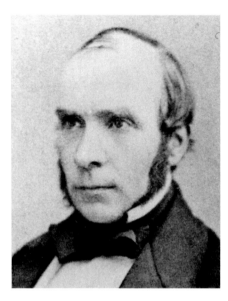

A pioneer anesthesiologist and a determined and patient collector of data, John Snow (1813–1858) pieced together evidence explaining the occurrence of cholera epidemics.

(sexually transmitted), skin diseases called "the itch" (transmitted by contact), and intestinal worms (fecal-oral transmission) as examples of different paths of transmission. This remarkable intellectual leap—the assumption that diseases may be transmitted through various routes, predated microbial evidence of the bacterial or viral causes of disease and anticipated the germ theory. Without it, Snow would not have been able to envision new routes of transmission so constructively.

He expressed his theory as follows: "Diseases which are communicated from person to person are caused by some material which passes from the sick to the healthy," and went on to define incubation as "the period which intervenes between the time when a morbid poison enters the system and the commencement of the illness which follows"; remarkably, he recognizes that "it is, in reality, a period of reproduction, as regards the morbid matter." The pathology of cholera suggested to Snow that in this case the "morbid" material is ingested through the mouth, multiplies in the gut, and is excreted with feces. Snow then explained how minute bits of a victim's excreta can contaminate food or water and enter the gut of another person, whereas close contact without exposure to excreta would not lead to infection. It seemed plausible to him that water can carry the cholera pathogen from one area to another when wells, streams, or pipes are contaminated by the sewage from households where cholera is present.

Snow proceeded to describe London outbreaks of cholera associated with a contaminated well on Thomas Street and a burst drain in Albion Terrace, culminating with an account of 89 deaths from cholera among persons drinking from the Broad Street pump. People who died had drunk from or brought water from the pump; those who had other sources of water (or consumed beer, like the workers at the adjacent brewery) did not get cholera (see the map on the facing page).

From the idea that contaminated wells could spread cholera, Snow expanded his hypothesis to include all water distribution systems, asserting that water companies that used contaminated sources could be spreading cholera to different areas of the city. Farr had prepared a tabulation of cholera deaths by London district and water company ("Report on the cholera of 1849"), and this report was cited and acknowledged by

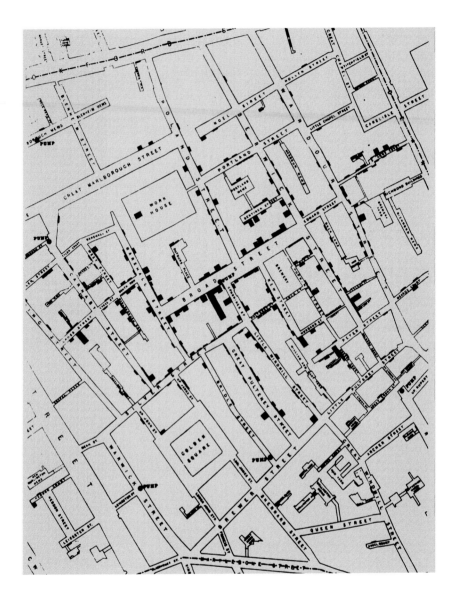

John Snow mapped the occurrence of cholera cases in these streets of London: a black bar for each death from August 19 to September 30, 1854, is placed in the situation of the house in which the fatal attack took place. He also marked the positions of the local water pumps. Snow deduced that water from the Broad Street pump was the source of cholera.

Snow, who grouped the districts by number of deaths per 10,000 inhabitants. The nine districts with the highest mortality were supplied by Southwark and Vauxhall Works (see the table on pages 36 and 37).

The epidemic of 1853 gave Snow a unique opportunity to further test his hypothesis and identify the specific water companies supplying conta-

Snow's Table III, "Showing the Mortality from Cholera, and the Water Supply, in the Districts of London, in 1849."

District	Population in the middle of 1849	Deaths from cholera	Deaths by cholera to 10,000 inhabits	Annual value of house and shop room to each person in £	Water supply
Rotherhithe	17,208	352	205	4.238	Southwark and Vauxhall Water Works, Kent Water Works, and Tidal Ditches
St. Olave, Southwark	19,278	349	181	4.559	Southwark and Vauxhall
St. George, Southwark	50,900	836	164	3.518	Southwark and Vauxhall, Lambeth
Bermondsey	45,500	734	161	3.077	Southwark and Vauxhall
St. Saviour, Southwark	35,227	539	153	5.291	Southwark and Vauxhall
Newington	63,074	907	144	3.788	Southwark and Vauxhall, Lambeth
Lambeth	134,768	1618	120	4.389	Southwark and Vauxhall, Lambeth
Wandsworth	48,446	484	100	4.839	Pump-wells, Southwark and Vauxhall, river Wandle
Camberwell	51,714	504	97	4.508	Southwark and Vauxhall, Lambeth
West London	28,829	429	96	7.454	New River
Bethnal Green	87,263	789	90	1.480	East London
Shoreditch	104,122	789	76	3.103	New River, East London
Greenwich	95,954	718	75	3.379	Kent
Poplar	44,103	313	71	7.360	East London
Westminster	64,109	437	68	4.189	Chelsea
Whitechapel	78,590	506	64	3.388	East London
St. Giles	54,062	285	53	5.635	New River
Stepney	106,988	501	47	3.319	East London
Chelsea	53,379	247	46	4.210	Chelsea
East London	43,495	182	45	4.823	New River
St. George's, East	47,334	199	42	4.753	East London
London City	55,816	207	38	17.676	New River
St. Martin	24,557	91	37	11.844	New River
Strand	44,254	156	35	7.374	New River
Holborn	46,134	161	35	5.883	New River
St. Luke	53,234	183	34	3.731	New River
Kensington (except Paddington)	110,491	260	33	5.070	West Middlesex, Chelsea, Grand Junction

Snow's Table III, Continued

District	Populaton in the middle of 1849	Deaths from cholera	Deaths by cholera to 10,000 inhabits	Annual value of house and shop room to each person in £	Water supply
Lewisham	32,299	96	30	4.824	Kent
Belgrave	37,918	105	28	8.875	Chelsea
Hackney	55,152	139	25	4.397	New River, East London
Islington	87,761	187	22	5.494	New River
St. Pancras	160,122	360	22	4.871	New River, Hampstead, West Middlesex
Clerkenwell	63,499	121	19	4.138	New River
Marylebone	153,960	261	17	7.586	West Middlesex
St. James, Westminster	36,426	57	16	12.669	Grand Junction, New River
Paddington	41,267	35	8	9.349	Grand Junction
Hampstead	11,572	9	8	5.804	Hampstead, West Middlesex
Hanover Square and May Fair	33,196	26	8	16.754	Grand Junction
London	2,280,282	14137	62	—	

minated water. Some districts received water from more than one water company, with no apparent pattern: "The pipes of each Company went down all the streets, and into nearly all the courts and alleys." Present-day epidemiologists would term Snow's next study a "natural experiment," because the researcher had not assigned subjects to the different water-supply companies; but Snow simply called it an experiment, and he seems to have grasped the main strengths of the well-conducted experiment with which circumstance had provided him:

The experiment, too, was on the grandest scale. No fewer than three hundred thousand people of both sexes, of every age and occupation, and of every rank and station, from gentlefolks down to the very poor, were divided into two groups without their choice, and, in most cases, without their knowledge; one group being supplied with water containing the sewage of London, and, amongst it, what ever might have come from the cholera patients, the other group having water quite free from such impurity. To turn this grand experiment to account, all that was required was to learn the supply of water to each individual house where a fatal attack of cholera might occur.

When the cholera returned in July of 1854, Snow was ready to conduct his study. Farr's General Register Office gave him the addresses of people dying of cholera in the districts served by more than one water company, and Snow then ascertained which water supply had been used by the cholera victims. After Farr saw the preliminary data, the registers of the study districts took over the ascertainment work begun by Snow. Snow, aware of the problems involved in determining the correct supplier (renters, for example, often did not know which company supplied their water), developed a chemical test to distinguish water supplies. He summarized the results he had gathered during the first seven weeks of the epidemic (ending August 26, 1854) in his Table IX. Mortality among persons consuming water supplied by Southwark and Vauxhall was ten times higher compared to the Lambeth Company and about five times higher than in the rest of London.

Snow's analysis was careful and thorough, and he courteously acknowledged the help given to him by Farr and the General Register Office. He cited other papers, reports, and literature, concluding with twelve

Snow's Table IX

	Number of houses	Deaths from cholera	Deaths per 10,000 houses
Southwark and Vauxhall Company	40,046	1,263	315
Lambeth Company	26,107	98	37
Rest of London	256,423	1,422	59

recommendations for the prevention of cholera and an expansion of his original hypothesis: if cholera can be transmitted through the water supply, perhaps other diseases are similarly transmitted and may be similarly prevented. He suggested that typhus, in particular, might be waterborne and therefore preventable. He turned out to be correct, in part. The Victorians did not recognize typhus and typhoid fever as distinct diseases; cases of either illness were classified as typhus. Later investigators confirmed that typhoid fever was waterborne, but typhus was proved to be transmitted by lice.

Others in the nineteenth century made great and equally important contributions to epidemiology, but John Snow wrote a description clearly proceeding through logical stages of evidence, from theory to case to experiment to implications. Snow did not consider himself to be an epidemiologist and certainly could not have anticipated the modern meaning of the word, but his work perfectly embodies the modern epidemiologic approach to a health problem.

Historians and philosophers of science can debate the exact nature of his contribution and his consciousness of its unique character. Did he see himself as the founder of a new discipline? What was the precise impact of his cholera work on the course of medicine? on the development of epidemiology? In the nineteenth and early twentieth centuries, epidemiology was propelled by discoveries in microbiology; the expression of a cohesive approach did not emerge until the 1930s and later. Those early epidemiologists who attempted to articulate their discipline's approach found in Snow a clear example, readily available, and they used this example in their teaching and writing to develop the profession.

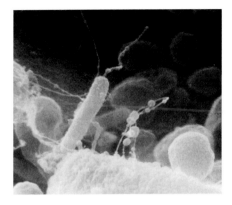

Snow's theory that a substance in the water supply caused cholera was later confirmed with the discovery of the cholera bacillus, *Vibrio cholerae*, shown here, magnified 25,000 times, attached to the intestinal lining in a mouse.

Florence Nightingale and Health Care Reform

FLORENCE Nightingale, another of Farr's collaborators, was likewise an epidemiologist without knowing it; she used statistics to measure health, identify causes of mortality, evaluate health services, and reform institutions. Although Nightingale is famous as "the lady with the lamp," nursing the wounded during the Crimean War, she was also an administrator

Florence Nightingale (1820–1910) was an ardent believer in the power of statistics to sway opinion, change policy, and institute reform.

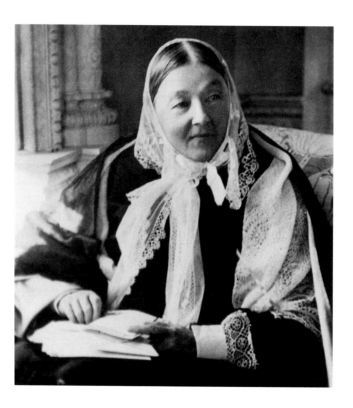

during that period and a theoretician the remainder of her life. She had studied mathematics with a tutor and then statistics through readings and correspondence with such men as Farr and Adolphe Quetelet, the Belgian statistician and expositor of sociological principles. Her experiences during the Crimean War convinced her that the health administration of the British Army needed a complete reform. Upon her return from the battlefield, she began organizing committees, assembling data, and preparing reports and hearings on how administrative inadequacies affected patients' health.

Nightingale was close to the British aristocracy; Lord Palmerston, Prime Minister at the conclusion of the Crimean War, had been her childhood friend. Her accomplishments in the Crimea increased her influence, and she found Queen Victoria responsive to many of her ideas. Meeting William Farr at a dinner party in 1856, she put him on her list of civilians to be appointed to the Army Sanitary Commission, and although his name was eventually dropped, Farr continued to work with Nightingale and to serve as an expert witness for the commission. Their analysis of mortality statistics for military and civilian men showed that even in peacetime, military mortality was higher than mortality among civilian males of similar age. This higher mortality they attributed to infectious diseases.

One of Florence Nightingale's "coxcombs," taken from her book *Notes on Matters Affecting the Health, Efficiency and Hospital Administration of the British Army*, published in 1858. The areas of the wedges, measured from the center, are proportional to the number of deaths in one of three categories: blue for deaths from contagious diseases such as cholera and typhus, red for deaths from wounds, and gray for deaths from all other causes. Nightingale intended to emphasize that deaths from contagious disease, which she believed could have been prevented through improved sanitary conditions, far outnumbered the deaths inflicted by combat.

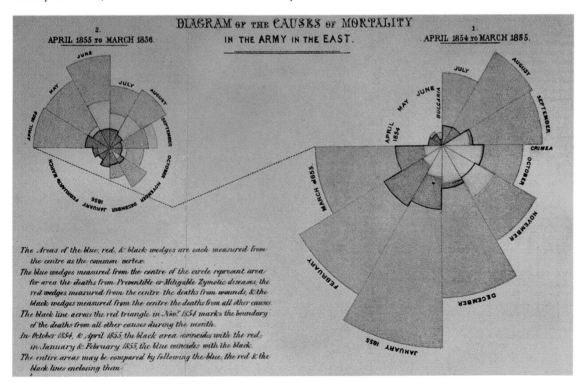

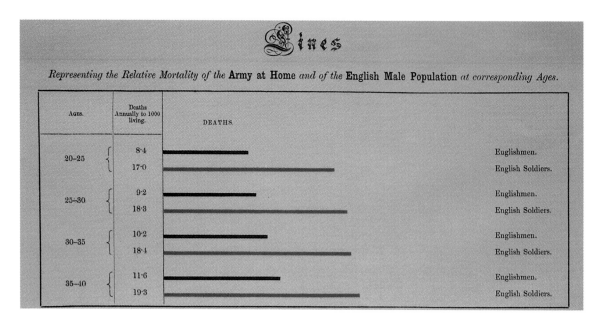

Florence Nightingale's statistics and charts helped to demonstrate that disease, poor food, and unsanitary conditions were killing English peacetime soldiers at rates in excess of those experienced by English civilians.

Nightingale published a thousand-page report, *Notes on Matters Affecting the Health, Efficiency and Hospital Administration of the British Army;* the commission published a separate report. One of Nightingale's particular contributions was the increased use of graphics to illustrate statistical relationships. She wanted statistical comparisons to have an impact on readers who might be too hurried to read text or tables, and for this purpose she had developed circular diagrams that she called her "coxcombs," illustrated on page 41. Nightingale's work not only had helped push the government to reform its administration of the British Army, but it also may be the first example of someone using health care data to affect governmental reforms in the interest of preventing death and disease.

Nightingale and Farr collaborated on many other projects; over four hundred of their letters exist. In 1858 Farr nominated Nightingale for admission to the Statistical Society, the first woman to be so admitted. In 1859, Nightingale drafted model hospital statistical forms using the General Register Office standard nosology (classification of diseases) to compare "relative mortalities of different hospitals." During the 1860s, Farr and Nightingale together studied hospital mortality data and mortality data of the British Army in India.

Working closely together for many years, the two seemed to influence each other. Nightingale chose to keep herself anonymous or in the background on many occasions, so it is especially difficult to assess her contribution to the use of statistics in epidemiology. Her application of statistics to health care administration and reform, however, was well ahead of her time, directly influencing the health of soldiers, hospital patients, and others. She did not think of herself as an epidemiologist, and modern epidemiologists have often overlooked her achievement; but the precedent set by her years of work, extensive reports, and diverse collaborations must have affected the people she worked with, as well as the public. It offered an example of the potential value of health statistics in the formation of public policy that has been more fully recognized in recent decades.

Epidemiology Emerges as a Separate Profession

IN 1850 the London Epidemiological Society, the first of its kind, was founded "with the specific purpose of determining the causes of and methods of preventing cholera and other 'epidemic diseases.' " The early use of the word *epidemiology* referred strictly to the study of epidemics, notably those of infectious origin. As late as the 1920s and 1930s, definitions emphasized epidemiology's concern with infectious disease—surely reflecting the excitement surrounding the great nineteenth- and early twentieth-century discoveries of infectious agents and the new understanding of disease transmission. The work of these microbiologists and bacteriologists channeled epidemiologic energies beyond searches for cause and transmission to means of prevention. By the 1950s and 1960s,

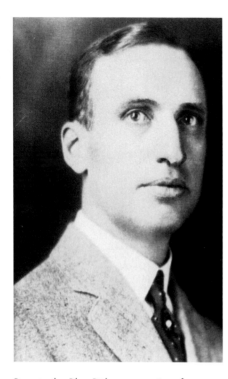

Born in the Blue Ridge mountains of Virginia, the seventh of eight children of a country physician, Wade Hampton Frost (1880–1938) became the first professor of epidemiology in the United States, and one of the first to formulate theoretical concepts of epidemiology.

epidemiologists preferred to define themselves in terms of the interaction between disease, humans, and the environment; the word *ecology* was commonly used in the definition of epidemiology. Since 1970, the emphasis on ecology has been replaced with an emphasis on distribution, occurrence, and pattern or variation. The earlier restriction to infectious illness is long gone, and the word disease is now used in its broadest sense to include any health-related outcome, including homicide.

From the founding of the London Epidemiological Society, the discipline slowly became recognized as a profession. Minnesota appointed the first state epidemiologist, W. H. Hill, in 1909, and the U.S. Public Health Service appointed its first epidemiologist, Allen W. Freeman, in 1915. The American Epidemiological Society was founded in 1927 with Charles V. Chapin as its first president, and the Epidemiology Section of the American Public Health Association was formed in 1929. Epidemiology grew out of the contemporary public health ("sanitary") movement and the hygiene movement, fueled by developments in microbiology and statistics. For example, today's *American Journal of Epidemiology* was founded in 1921 as the *American Journal of Hygiene.*

At the turn of the century, most epidemiologists were physicians who investigated the mysteries of infectious diseases. Wade Hampton Frost, the first American professor of epidemiology, studied the high prevalence of typhoid in Washington, D.C., the 1916 epidemic of poliomyelitis, and the 1918 epidemic of influenza. After assuming his professorship at the Johns Hopkins School of Hygiene and Public Health in 1921, Frost devoted special efforts to describing the epidemiologic approach and to consciously developing a model of epidemiology. In 1927 he wrote a theoretical paper, "Epidemiology," which used Snow's work as an example of the discipline. In his first few pages he restricted the definition to infectious diseases, but he went on to describe the logical process that characterizes epidemiology:

> In collecting facts about the distribution of disease, the purpose in view is always to arrive at a better understanding of its nature, sources, means of spread, and eventually its control. This

implies that the facts must be related to each other in such an orderly way as to establish a theory or philosophy of the disease; and, as this theory must be consistent with all the accepted principles of the broader natural philosophy into which it is fitted, epidemiology must come into relation here with the whole field of natural science, but more especially that of biology. The opinion is more or less prevalent that inferences based upon epidemiological argument cannot be truly conclusive, because the evidence is purely circumstantial. Such opinion has frequently failed to take account of the whole mass of evidence, and to follow the argument which is necessarily built up step-by-step in a somewhat complex and perhaps tedious way. Given sufficient scope and accuracy of observations, a conclusion as to the nature and spread of a disease may often be established quite firmly by circumstantial evidence well in advance of experimental confirmation. Moreover, many problems of disease transmission which are highly important from the standpoint of prevention, are such that can be solved only by investigations of this kind.

When Frost used phrases like "epidemiological argument," he no longer restricted discussion to the type of disease being studied, but characterized the science of epidemiology by the type of argument or inquiry used and its intellectual approach. In Frost's formulation, the discipline was becoming less the study of infectious diseases and more a method or thought process, which others would be able to apply to the study of noninfectious diseases.

Joseph Goldberger's Investigation of Diet and Disease

EPIDEMIOLOGISTS were already studying such diseases, even if unintentionally. In March 1914 Dr. Joseph Goldberger, an accomplished epidemiologist who had worked with infectious diseases only (typhus, measles, diphtheria, and others), was assigned by the U.S. Surgeon Gen-

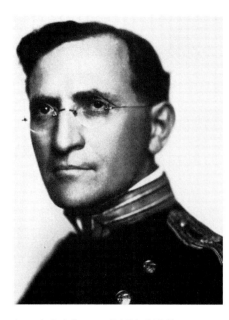

Joseph Goldberger (1874–1929), wearing the uniform of the U.S. Public Health Service. Goldberger was assigned the task of solving the pellagra epidemic; in doing so, he expanded the scope of epidemiology to include noninfectious diseases.

eral to take charge of the pellagra studies of the U.S. Public Health Service. Pellagra was first reported in the United States in 1863, but by 1912 there may have been 25,000 cases in the country with a case fatality rate of 40 percent. Doctors called pellagra the disease of the three "D's"—dermatitis, dementia, and diarrhea. The skin became reddened, scaly, crusty, and infected; sores developed in the mouth, tongue, lip, and bowel. Patients became demented and often were committed to insane asylums.

The Thompson-McFadden Pellagra Commission had concluded in 1913 that "pellagra is in all probability a specific infectious disease communicable from person to person by means at present unknown"; it was natural to assign an epidemiologist to investigate this new epidemic. Three months after Goldberger accepted charge of the pellagra investigation, he wrote his first paper, asserting that pellagra was not infectious. He based his conclusion on three observations regarding the pattern of pellagra occurrence: no case had ever been reported among the doctors, nurses, or attendants who cared for pellagra patients; the disease occurred mainly in rural areas; and only poor people appeared to get pellagra. If the disease was contagious it should have occasionally appeared in caretakers, urban areas, or among the upper classes.

Goldberger initiated a wide range of studies to disprove the infectious disease hypothesis and to support his hypothesis that pellagra was related to diet. To demonstrate that pellagra was noninfectious, he and his wife and colleagues experimented on themselves. They injected themselves with, or swallowed, preparations of pellagra patients' blood, sputum, skin, urine, and feces in a series of "filth parties" (as he called them). His wife volunteered to represent women and described her experiences in the May 21, 1929, edition of the *New York Times*. Goldberger and his colleagues conducted seven "filth parties" and concluded, "If anyone can get pellagra that way, we three should certainly have it good and hard."

At this juncture, Goldberger paved the way for noninfectious disease epidemiology. Knowing that pellagra was not infectious, he took methods that had been used to discover the causes of infectious diseases alone and applied them to the problem of pellagra.

Goldberger conducted experiments in two orphanages showing that a diet supplemented with milk, eggs, meat, beans, and peas resulted in a decreased incidence of pellagra. He conducted the reverse type of experiment, producing pellagra in healthy prisoners in Rankin Prison Farm in Mississippi by confining them to a diet of biscuits, mush, grits, gravy, syrup, coffee, sugar, cornbread, collards, and sweet potatoes. In the orphanage studies he compared the incidence of pellagra before and after dietary changes. In the prison study, two groups of men were assigned to separate diets, one standard prison fare, the other the experimental diet that produced pellagra. (The prison farm experiment is not, of course, ethical by today's standards, and modern epidemiologists no longer conduct experiments with the objective of producing disease in humans.)

Goldberger continued his research on pellagra for many years. With Edgar Sydenstricker, he conducted community surveys to analyze the in-

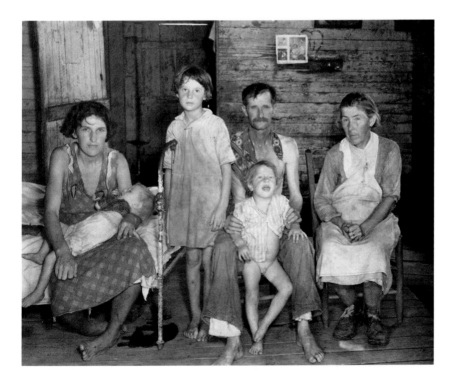

Rural poverty in the South, as portrayed in this photograph by Walker Evans, resulted in the limited diets that led to pellagra.

fluence of employment, income, and other economic factors on the incidence of pellagra. He also instigated animal studies to identify the factors responsible for pellagra. Before Goldberger's death in 1929 he had postulated that "water soluble B" vitamin included a heat-sensitive, pellagra-preventive factor. In 1937 C. A. Elvehjem demonstrated that nicotinic acid (niacin) was the antipellagra factor.

The Goldberger research is another example of epidemiologic methods being used to prevent or control an epidemic well before the pathogenic or biochemical cause was identified. As early as 1916 Goldberger had demonstrated the role of diet in preventing or causing pellagra. Two decades later, the precise dietary deficiency was identified. In the inter-

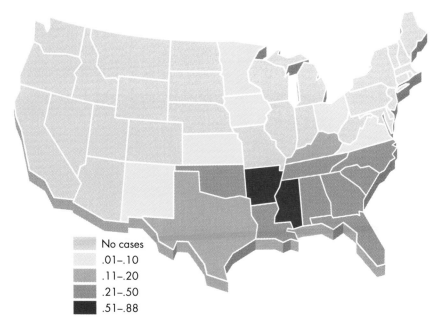

No cases
.01–.10
.11–.20
.21–.50
.51–.88

Pellagra was concentrated in the southeast of the United States with its large numbers of poor subsisting on corn-based diets. This map describes the incidence of pellagra in men drafted into the U.S. Army during World War I by state of home residence. Statistics on physical characteristics of over 2 million draftees were compiled and published in a 1920 government report, *Defects Found in Drafted Men*.

vening twenty years, thousands of cases of pellagra were treatable because of Goldberger's work, which perhaps also spurred laboratory efforts to identify niacin, the vitamin whose deficiency results in pellagra. Since this discovery, pellagra has been eliminated in the United States because common foods such as flour, bread, and breakfast cereals are supplemented with niacin. Goldberger, nominated for the Nobel Prize five times, never received it.

Epidemiology continues to expand its scope beyond the original tasks of tracking and halting infectious epidemics. In the chapters to come we follow epidemiology into the present by focusing on a number of issues that not only occupy modern epidemiologists, but have also, in effect, redefined the discipline. Epidemiologic contributions to the understanding of lung and other cancers, for example, began in the 1950s and continue to expand, simultaneously widening the definition of epidemiology. Epidemiologic attention to the "epidemic" of heart disease has been responsible for dramatic changes in the incidence of heart disease, and for the development of new methods of treatment. Pharmacology, therapy evaluation, occupational and environmental health have all used epidemiologic approaches, forcing the growth of that discipline. The history of epidemiology does not end with this chapter. In a field that is rapidly changing and growing, history is being written every day.

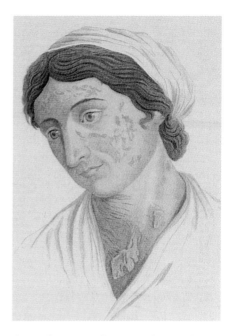

This early nineteenth century drawing by G. L. Alibert portrays the reddening and thickening of the skin seen in the victims of pellagra.

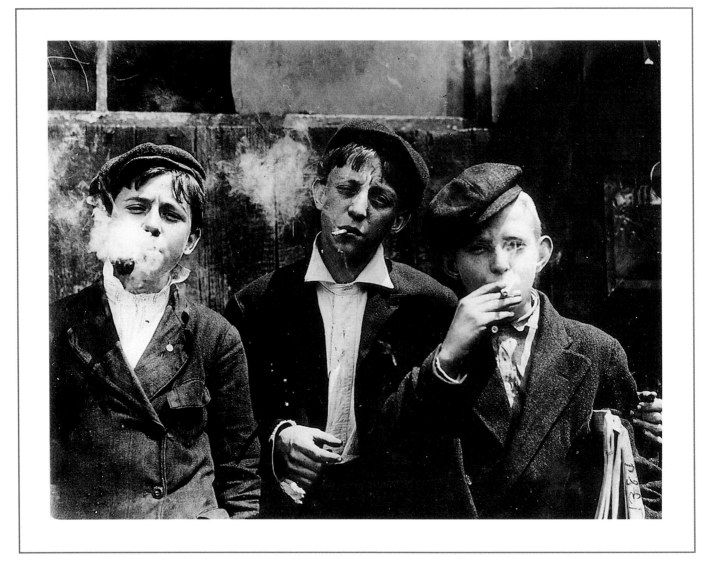

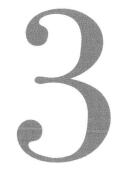

Lung Cancer: New Methods of Studying Disease

A PHOTOGRAPH from 1910 shows several newsboys puffing on cigarettes. Smoking began to grow in popularity early in this century, and the widespread adoption of the habit was eventually reflected in rising lung cancer rates.

Cancer was described long ago by the ancient Egyptians and Greeks. Hippocrates originated the term carcinoma from *karkinos* (crab); ancient Greeks saw cancer as crablike in its spread over the body and in its persistence. A passage attributed both to Hippocrates and to Paulus of Aegina describes a tumor:

> It appears at length with turgid veins shooting out from it, so as to resemble the figure of a crab; or as others say, becomes like a crab: where it has once got, it is scarcely possible to drive it away.

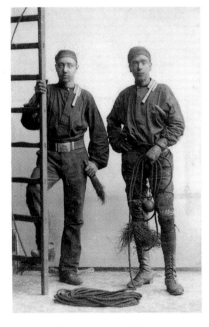

For several hundred years chimney sweeps were known to have high rates of scrotal cancer, which was called "the soot wart" in recognition of its presumed association with exposure to soot.

Cancer was regarded as a dread and mysterious disease. It could arise in any part of the body, it could spread to other parts of the body, it appeared to be incurable—and more strangely yet, it did not spread to other people. Even if it showed some tendencies to recur in families, it did not threaten the health of caregivers or other household members.

Epidemics of contagious diseases such as syphilis, cholera, or plague historically incited more fear than did cancer, but as infectious diseases became controlled in modern times through improved sanitation, vaccination, and antibiotics, medical attention turned toward cancer and heart disease, major causes of mortality in the twentieth-century United States and Europe. The story of cancer epidemiology thus encompasses the transition that took place in the discipline as a whole from the 1950s onward. Could the epidemiologic method, developed in response to infectious disease models, be applied to the study of cancer?

In eighteenth-century England, chimney sweeps called scrotal cancer "the soot wart," intuitively identifying soot as the cause of their cancer. The British physician Percival Pott, in 1775, described its rampant occurrence among these boys, inferring that something in their work explained the remarkable toll from scrotal cancer. Ludwig Rehn, in 1895, first reported an association between bladder cancer and work with aniline dyes. F. H. Harting and W. Hesse, in 1879, showed that 75 percent of deaths among miners of silver, cobalt, and uranium were due to lung cancer. These early observations of cancers associated with occupational exposure paved the way for the extensive work in occupational and environmental epidemiology of the last few decades, but they also implicated a confusingly wide variety of exposures as increasing one's risk of cancer. Bernardino Ramazzini first noticed the high incidence of breast cancer among nuns in 1700; he attributed their risk to celibacy. His observation of an association between convent life and breast cancer was accurate, but it was lack of childbearing that explained the nuns' high risk. Pertinent observations, clearly, were open to misinterpretation.

"Cures" for cancer were advertised, sold, and proclaimed in the nineteenth and twentieth centuries; "discoverers" of the cause of cancer were rife. In 1926 the Nobel Prize was awarded to Johannes Fibiger, a Danish pathologist, for discovering the "cause" of stomach cancer, which he identified as the nematode *Spiroptera carcinoma*. In assigning his award the committee declared, "Fibiger was the first . . . to succeed in lifting with a sure hand a corner of the veil which hid from us the etiology of this disease." Fibiger had appeared to demonstrate that the parasite caused stomach tumors in rats. In fact, dietary deficiencies in the rat feed, combined with misreading of the tissue slides, explained his erroneous findings, as was shown in 1937 and 1952 by scientists attempting to replicate Fibiger's work. Contemporary with Fibiger, however, were efforts to prove that viruses cause cancer and that tar causes cancer—two hypotheses that later research would support. Accurate and inaccurate observations stood side by side, therefore, equally difficult to interpret in a scientific world where genetics and virology had not yet been substantially developed.

Despite the long history of observations, understanding of cancer biology did not compare to medical understanding of infectious disease. The variety of observations pointed in different directions as to probable causes—indeed, they challenged what was meant by the word "cause." If, for example, uranium miners died of lung cancer and cigarette smokers also showed a high incidence of that disease, what common factor was "causing" the lung cancer? Epidemiologists had to revise their concept of causality to explore cancer epidemiology (and other diseases with multiple causes). How the epidemiologic methods, concepts, and techniques

The cover of a cartoon booklet from the 1950s, warning the public of the signs of cancer.

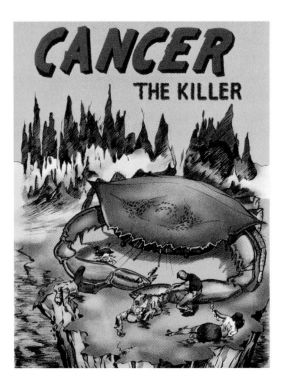

used to study infectious diseases evolved in response to the challenge of cancer is a process well illustrated by the story of cigarette smoking and lung cancer.

Early Observations on Tobacco and Cancer

THE association between tobacco use and cancer was noted as early as 1761 (when John Hill described cases of nasal cancer among snuff users) and 1795 (when Samuel von Sömmerring pointed to a possible connection between lip cancer and pipe smoking). In 1920, A. C. Broders published a study comparing 537 male lip cancer patients to 500 men without lip cancer: he noted a higher number of pipe smokers in the lip cancer group than in the healthy men (78 percent of lip cancer patients smoked pipes, compared to 38 percent of healthy men). In a 1928 study of the habits, characteristics, and environment of people with and without cancer, Herbert Lombard and Carl Doering examined tobacco use. Although they had no lung cancer cases in their sample, they nonetheless found 47.3 percent of cancer cases to have been heavy smokers, compared to 20 percent among their controls, and interpreted the findings to suggest "that heavy smoking has some relation to cancer in general." In 1938, Raymond Pearl published a life table, a table describing the mortality and survival of a group of individuals over a period of time derived from records of 6,813 white men categorized into three groups: nonsmokers, moderate smokers, and heavy smokers. The table and the survival curves showed an association between smoking and decreased longevity, and the author concluded that "the smoking of tobacco was statistically associated with an impair-

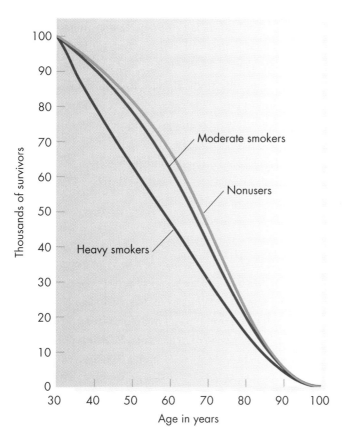

In 1938 Raymond Pearl graphed the percentages surviving at each age for heavy smokers, moderate smokers, and nonsmokers. At each age, heavy smokers had more deaths (lower survivorship) than did moderate smokers and nonsmokers.

ment of life duration, and the amount or degree of this impairment increased as the habitual amount of smoking increased."

Much of epidemiology involves either the recognition of a new disease or syndrome, or the recognition of an increase in a known disease. Occasional increases in rare diseases may be due to chance fluctuation; slight increases may be a result of changes in case detection or diagnosis. At the turn of the century, lung cancer was rare among cancers and among causes of death in the United States—it wasn't even on the list of seven main types of cancer considered in Lombard and Doering's 1928 research. By the 1930s and 1940s, physicians had begun writing about an "apparent" increase in lung cancer, wondering whether it was real or merely an artifact of better diagnosis and reporting. Mortality statistics, autopsy findings, and physician observations suggested that lung cancer was indeed more common than it had been, but medical authorities were reluctant to acknowledge the epidemic increase of lung cancer. The *British Medical Journal* of 1942 stated, "It is doubtful whether the higher incidence of cancer of the lung observed in recent years is real or only apparent," and the Medical Research Council of Great Britain report of 1948–50 reiterated, "the increase may, of course, be only apparent."

In Britain, the percentage of lung cancer among cancer deaths rose from 1.5 in 1920 to 19.7 in 1947. In Connecticut, the age-adjusted incidence of lung cancer among males rose from 9.7 per 1,000 in 1935–9 to 20.6 per 1,000 in 1945–9 and 31.1 per 1,000 in 1950–4. Diagnostic

(Facing Page) Lung cancer is an example of a carcinoma, a cancer that develops in the epithelial cells that form the linings of body cavities. Lung cancer arises in the epithelial cells lining the bronchial tubes. Normally there are two layers of epithelial cells (columnar and basal) resting on a layer of small, round cells called the basement membrane (1). One of smoking's first effects on the normal bronchial tube lining is an increase in the number of basal cells (2). The cells become squamous, or flattened (3), then develop the atypical nuclei of cancer cells (4). The abnormal cells eventually break through the basement membrane, spreading the cancer through the lungs and to the rest of the body.

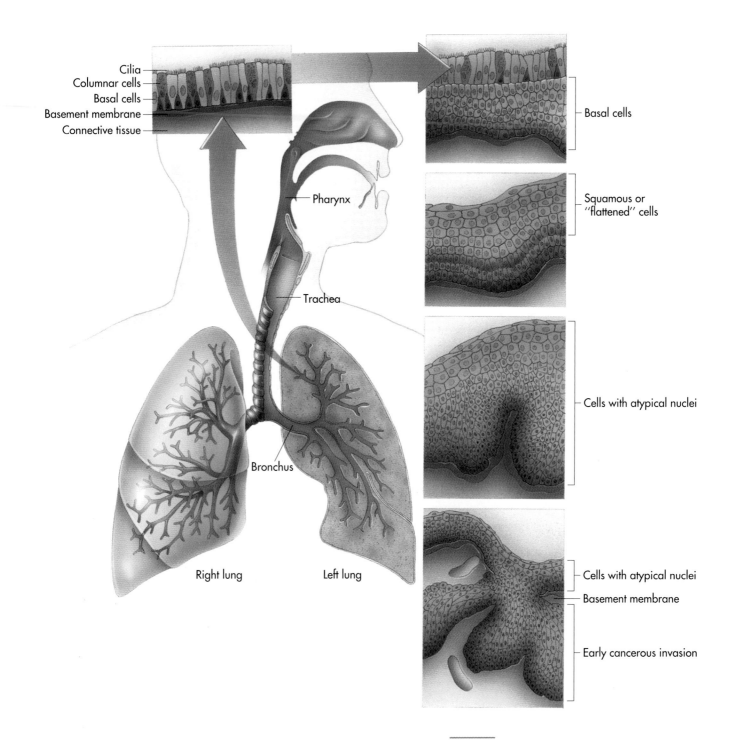

Cilia
Columnar cells
Basal cells
Basement membrane
Connective tissue

Basal cells

Squamous or "flattened" cells

Cells with atypical nuclei

Cells with atypical nuclei
Basement membrane
Early cancerous invasion

Pharynx

Trachea

Bronchus

Right lung

Left lung

Marlene Dietrich was just one of many glamorous celebrities who smoked. Before much was known about the hazards of smoking, cigarettes seemed glamorous too.

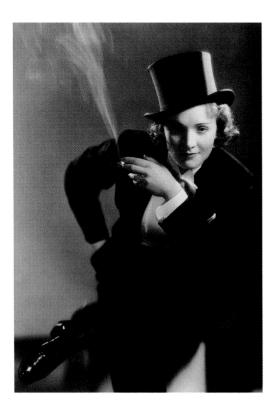

methods had improved by the 1940s and 1950s, and greater life expectancy increased one's chance of developing cancer (generally speaking, a disease of advancing age). But these facts could not explain the magnitude of the increase in lung cancer. In 1952, the *Lancet* wrote, "There is little doubt that the increase is both real and numerically important."

A New Study Design to Describe the Relationship Between Smoking and Lung Cancer

IN 1950 a medical student, Ernst Wynder, and a professor of surgery, Evart Graham, described 684 cases of bronchiogenic carcinoma in the United States. Almost simultaneously Richard Doll and Bradford Hill published their study of 709 cases of lung carcinoma patients in Great Britain. Both studies made new use of a method that offered immediate results, called the case-control method. The studies compared individuals with the disease to controls (people without the disease) to see if an exposure or risk factor—in this instance, tobacco smoking—was the same or different in each group.

The epidemiologic study of cancer posed several difficulties: cancer was relatively rare (31 deaths per 1,000 in 1950–4, about 3 percent of the population), and it appeared to develop slowly over twenty to thirty years. It would take many years and large study sample sizes to follow groups of smokers and nonsmokers and measure their rates of lung cancer. A study that began in 1950 might not produce results until 1970 or 1980. A case-control study circumvents these problems by studying people who already have the disease (in our examples, they were diagnosed in the early 1950s) and collecting information about exposures in the past (the 1920s or 1930s). It allowed epidemiologists to collect information regarding the hypothesis that an increase in smoking was the cause of the increase in lung cancer.

The studies of Wynder and Graham and of Doll and Hill both found more smokers among the lung cancer patients than among the control group. Both pairs of authors were cautious in their conclusions, Wynder and Graham writing that "the data suggest, although they do not establish, a causal relation between cigarette and pipe smoking and cancer of the lung and lip, respectively." Doll and Hill wrote, "Taken as a whole, the lung-carcinoma patients had begun to smoke earlier and had continued for longer than the controls, but the differences were very small and not statistically significant."

With hindsight we know that these early studies did not show the full effect of smoking on lung cancer because they used hospital populations for controls—often specifically those patients with pulmonary ailments. The hospitalized controls were sick with other diseases, many of which (we now know) are caused or exacerbated by cigarette smoking. The hospital controls probably included a higher proportion of smokers than would be found in the general population, so the contrast in smoking history between lung cancer patients and hospitalized patients (without lung

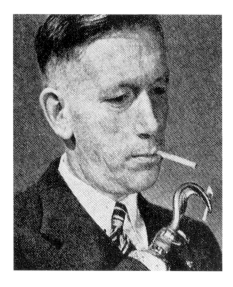

Despite the growing scientific discussion of the effect of smoking on lung cancer, the general public considered smoking to be an acceptable social habit. As late as 1946, even the American Medical Association used the photo of a man smoking to illustrate the complete adjustment of a man to his prosthetic hand—his artificial hand was so good that he could lead a normal life, and smoke again!

cancer) was less than the contrast between lung cancer patients and the general population. As a consequence, the studies underestimated the true risk associated with lung cancer. Nevertheless, they found considerable differences between the two groups and generated much controversy.

One area of technical controversy concerned how to estimate relative risk using case-control data. When John Snow did his analysis of cholera deaths (described in Chapter 2), he was able to compute the number of deaths among people using different water companies; comparing the rates, he could estimate the relative risk of contracting cholera as ten times higher among people served by one particular water company than among other Londoners. Snow could calculate rates because the entire population of his "natural experiment" was characterized by exposure (all had some water supply) and the cholera deaths could be assigned to the different exposure groups (according to supplying water company). In case-control studies, however, one does not usually know very much about the general population. When the Wynder and Graham and the Doll and Hill papers were published, readers could see that the proportions of smokers were different in the case and control groups, but the authors could not calculate how much the risk of lung cancer was increased by smoking.

To estimate the risk of lung cancer, one needs to define the number of people at risk (the denominator) and the number of people who develop lung cancer (the numerator). To estimate the risk associated with smoking, one needs to know the number of smokers, the number of nonsmok-

Wynder and Graham's Data

	Male lung cancer patients	Male patients, other diseases
Smokers	584 (96.5%)	575 (73.7%)
Nonsmokers	21	205
	605	780

Doll and Hill's Data

	Male lung cancer patients	Male patients, other diseases
Smokers	647 (99.7%)	622 (95.8%)
Nonsmokers	2	27
	649	649

Calculating Odds Ratios

The odds ratio is simple to calculate. The investigator begins by plugging numbers for a, b, c, and d in a two-by-two table:

	Cases	Controls
Exposed to suspect carcinogen	a	b
Not exposed	c	d
	a+c	b+d

Then an elementary calculation is performed: cells a and d are multiplied and that number is divided by the product of b and c. Using Wynder and Graham's figures, the result is

$$OR = \frac{584\,(205)}{575\,(21)} = 9.76$$

Using Doll and Hill's figures, the result is

$$OR = \frac{647\,(27)}{622\,(2)} = 14.04$$

Jerome Cornfield suggested using the odds ratio to estimate risk in 1951, one year after Wynder and Graham's and Doll and Hill's papers appeared. The odds ratio shows more clearly than the original data (presented in the tables on the opposite page) how much smoking increases the risk of lung cancer. ●

ers (the two denominators), and the number of cases of lung cancer occurring in each group (the two numerators). These fractions can then be compared to estimate the relative risk.

In a case-control study, denominator data are not available, but the statistician Jerome Cornfield, in 1951, suggested using the cross-products or odds ratio as an estimate of relative risk. Comparing lung cancer patients to controls with respect to smoking histories, one can present the data in a two-by-two table as shown on the previous page. The cross-products (odds ratio) of the table cells are produced by the method illustrated in the box on this page: one multiplies the cells a and d and divides that number by the product of cells b and c. If the cases are representative of the population of diseased people, the controls representative of the gen-

Interpreting a Low Odds Ratio

While a high relative risk or odds ratio is important in establishing that an exposure causes a given disease, lower relative risks can be important as well. For example, a high relative risk of 20 for smokers and lung cancer would mean that smokers are 20 times more likely than nonsmokers to develop lung cancer, a crucial fact in understanding the causal relationship between smoking and lung cancer. The much lower relative risk of 1.2 associated with passive smoking (inhaling smoke from other people's cigarettes in the home or workplace, in restaurants or waiting rooms) and lung cancer is less dramatic evidence for a causal relationship, but is still important because passive smoking may affect many more people. A relative risk of 1.2 means that passive smoking increases one's risk of lung cancer by 20 percent. To an individual a 20-percent increase in low risk—say, from a probability of 1.0 in a 1,000 to 1.2 in 1,000—may not substantially change the overall level of risk. But in the case of passive smoking, since large segments of the population can be exposed to passive smoke, a 20-percent increase in risk can result in a substantial increase in the number of people with cancer whose disease can be *attributable* to passive smoking. Low *relative* risks can produce high *attributable* risks—large numbers of affected people—and thus have important consequences for public health. •

eral population, and the incidence of disease low, the odds ratio (OR) of a case-control study approximates relative risk.

Using the data collected in the work done by Wynder and Graham and by Doll and Hill, we can calculate odds ratios for their studies. Wynder and Graham's data show an OR of 9.8, while the figures collected by Doll and Hill produce an OR of 14.0. These data suggest that cigarette smokers are 10 to 14 times more likely to develop lung cancer than are nonsmokers. (As we mentioned earlier, the actual risk is somewhat higher when nonhospital controls are used.)

A Challenge to Epidemiologic Thinking

LUNG cancer was profoundly different from the diseases that had previously been studied by epidemiologists. It appeared to develop twenty, thirty, or even forty years after the initial exposure; in other words, it showed a long latency period. Not everyone who smoked developed lung cancer, and some people developed lung cancer who had never smoked. Evidence from case-control studies was not convincing by itself, partly because the study design was new and unfamiliar and partly because the design has some intrinsic weaknesses. In a case-control study, for example, one cannot always establish the temporality of events—that is, whether smoking preceded lung cancer or whether a tendency toward lung cancer led one to smoke. Thus the renowned statistician R. A. Fisher (himself a smoker) suggested that individuals can be genetically predisposed to smoking and to lung cancer. Further research—studies that went beyond the case-control method—was needed to describe the health effects of smoking.

Investigators turned to another type of study, the cohort study (sometimes called prospective or follow-up), which follows a group of people for many years to see who develops a given disease. The term prospective refers to the fact that data are collected as events happen; retrospective studies, in contrast, collect data from records or patients' recall, *after* events have happened. The term follow-up means that the people are seen more than once, and the term cohort refers to a group of people who enter an observation period at similar points in time. Thus, it is possible to reconstruct a cohort historically and have a retrospective cohort study by selecting a group of people and finding out what happened to them in the past.

A prospective, follow-up study published in 1954 by E. Cuyler Hammond and Daniel Horn described mortality in 187,766 men aged 50 to 69 who had been followed for three years. The men were recruited by volunteers of the American Cancer Society in 394 counties in New Jersey, Pennsylvania, New York, Michigan, Illinois, Wisconsin, Minnesota, Iowa,

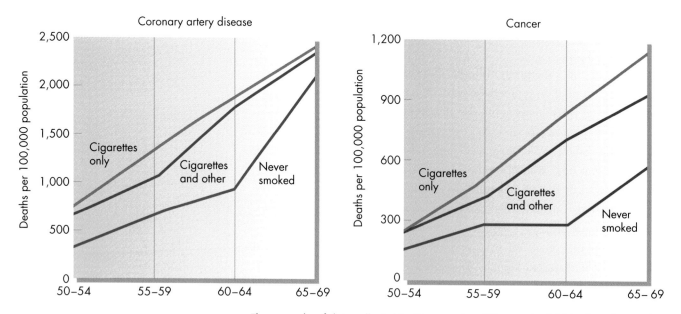

These graphs of data collected by Hammond and Horn in the 1950s show that smokers had higher numbers of deaths from coronary artery disease at all ages, as well as higher numbers of cancer deaths. Such data increased concern about the hazards of smoking, but also raised questions about causality: How could one activity, smoking, cause increases in two apparently unrelated diseases?

and California. The volunteers administered a questionnaire to find out the men's smoking habits, then contacted them at yearly intervals. As the subjects died, the study recorded each cause of death. This research added fuel to the controversy, because it showed an increased number of deaths from *all* causes among smokers—from coronary artery disease, for example, as well as from all cancers. Data from such a large prospective study were impressive, but the association between smoking and all mortality, including that from noncancer causes, seemed to confuse the issue. How could one agent cause or increase the risk of so many different diseases? Was this biologically plausible?

During the revolution in microbiology that took place at the turn of the century, two microbiologists had developed criteria for determining whether a given pathogen was the cause of a particular disease. The German anatomist and pathologist Jakob Henle first set forth his ideas in 1840, and his countryman Robert Koch revised them in 1884 and 1890, a period when pathogens were being discovered at the rate of one or two a year. To establish that a pathogen indeed caused a disease, the pathogen should cause *only* that disease, and no other pathogen should cause the disease. These were the Henle-Koch postulates, and they embodied much of epidemiologic thinking about causality.

Critics of the smoking and lung cancer research charged that if smoking was associated with increased mortality from several diseases, it could not be a true cause of lung cancer according to the Henle-Koch postulates. Other factors such as air pollution or mining, moreover, appeared to increase the risk of lung cancer, so smoking wasn't a necessary cause of lung cancer. In addition to debating the scientific merits of the smoking/lung cancer hypothesis, therefore, the health community began to debate the epidemiologic concept of causality—when is a factor a "cause" of disease? The Henle-Koch postulates had proved inadequate in addressing the causes of chronic and noninfectious diseases.

In the late 1950s, Abraham Lilienfeld, Jacob Yerushalmy, Phillip Sartwell, and A. Bradford Hill began adapting the concepts of causality to the study of chronic diseases. Hill suggested that the following be considered when drawing conclusions about a relationship between two variables and deciding whether there is true causation or mere association:

- *Strength of association:* How strong is the association between the exposure and disease? Usually expressed as relative risk or an odds ratio, the farther the risk from the number one, the stronger the association.
- *Consistency:* Is the association observed by different researchers in different conditions, circumstances, places, or times?
- *Specificity:* Is the cause usually found when the disease is present? Does the disease usually result when the cause is present?

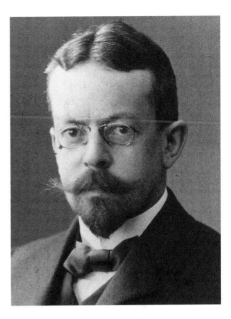

Jakob Henle (1809–1885) was the first to put forth postulates for considering the pathogens that cause disease.

The noted microbiologist Robert Koch (1843–1910) was the first to isolate anthrax bacteria, as well as the tuberculosis bacillus. He modified Henle's postulates, now called the Koch-Henle postulates or, more commonly, Koch's postulates.

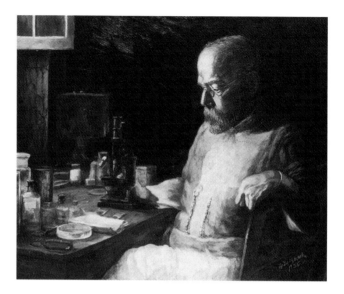

- *Relationship in time:* Does the exposure (or causal factor) precede the disease or outcome?
- *Biological gradient:* Does more exposure (higher amounts per unit time or longer duration of time exposed) lead to more severe disease or increased incidence of disease?
- *Biological plausibility:* Is the observed association consistent with biological ideas about the disease process?
- *Coherence of the evidence:* Does the entire set of observations fit together?
- *Experiment:* Does removal of the exposure result in a change in disease frequency? How does treatment affect different groups in a randomized trial?
- *Reasoning by analogy:* Are there similar known patterns of cause and effect found in other areas of epidemiology?

These concepts, put forth by Hill in 1965, were never intended to be formalized into a checklist of criteria; he clearly pointed out situations that would be exceptions to each of these concepts. For example, when writing about consistency of associations, he said, "There will be occasions when repetition is absent or impossible and yet we should not hesitate to draw conclusions." He gave as examples occupational studies of the 1920s and 1930s showing an association between nickel mining and nasal cancer in men who worked in the plant before 1923 (before certain changes in the refining process). No cases occurred after 1923, and Hill, in 1964, considered the absence of reoccurrence to be strong evidence implicating the abandoned refining process as a cause of nasal cancer. It is hard to say, thirty years later, whether present-day epidemiologists would rely on a single study. Replication of study results is part of the scientific process, but Hill had the foresight to realize that exceptions might arise. He concluded his suggestions with a discussion of common sense and its role in judging causality. The principles described by Bradford Hill remain basic guidelines in assessing a body of literature with respect to causality.

The evidence against cigarette smoking accumulated. By 1959 the U.S. Surgeon General had stated, "The weight of evidence at present implicates smoking as the principal etiological factor in the increased incidence of lung cancer." In 1964, the Surgeon General released *Smoking and Health*, a report that concluded, "Smoking is causally related to lung cancer." Early in their report, the authors discussed their bases for judgment, the "criteria of the epidemiologic method," and causality—how they decided if a relationship was causal, and what they meant by the word "cause." The report cited the magnitude of effect (strength of association) as far outweighing all other factors in its consideration of the evidence. The second point cited was the presence of a dose-response relationship: "the risk of developing lung cancer increases with duration of smoking and the number of cigarettes smoked per day."

The Surgeon General's report may be the first time that a discussion of the epidemiologic method and the concept of causality introduced a major report on a U.S. public health problem. It tacitly acknowledged that the epidemiologic method is appropriate and essential in addressing public health issues, that it is not restricted to problems of infectious diseases, and that epidemiologic evidence counts importantly in the formation of public policy. Further, it expanded the debate over causality, legitimizing a new interpretation and challenging the profession to con-

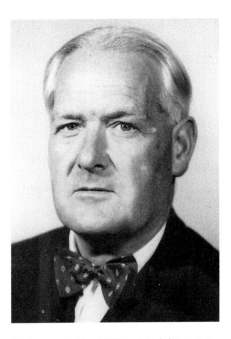

Sir Austin Bradford Hill, a British biostatistician who wrote with clarity and common sense, spreading the use of epidemiologic principles. He first wrote his ideas in the 1930s in a series of papers for the British medical journal *The Lancet*. In 1965 he summarized contemporary thinking on causality in a discussion of points to consider when assessing causality, still known as the "Bradford Hill criteria."

It takes twenty to thirty years, or longer, to develop lung cancer. Although cigarette smoking was nearing its peak in 1950, the lung cancer epidemic did not peak until 1980 or thereafter. In 1950 it was not clear that lung cancer mortality would truly follow the trends in cigarette consumption, but with hindsight we can see that it did.

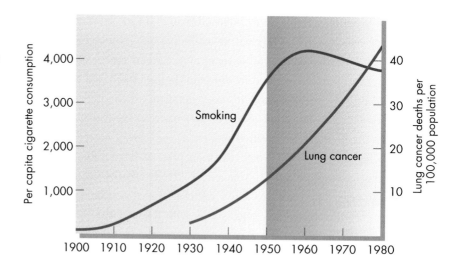

tinue rethinking what can be labeled the "cause" of a disease and what criteria are appropriate for assigning this label.

The epidemic increase in lung cancer could be explained by increased cigarette smoking. In the process of clarifying the relationship between smoking and lung cancer, epidemiologists also eventually documented increased risks of laryngeal, oral, esophageal, bladder, pancreatic, and renal cancers associated with cigarette smoking. Cigarette smoking was identified as a major cause of heart disease mortality, stroke, and peripheral vascular disease, as well as a cause of chronic bronchitis and emphysema and a factor in low-birthweight babies and unsuccessful pregnancies. The National Center for Health Statistics attributed 150,000 deaths to smoking in 1965. Forty-two percent of heart disease deaths in 1965 among males aged 35 to 64 could be attributed to cigarette smoking, as could 86 percent of all lung cancer deaths in males.

After 1964, epidemiologists became increasingly occupied with describing the health effects of smoking. While the tobacco industry and policymakers continued to debate the implications of scientific findings, farsighted epidemiologists turned their attention to disease prevention and health promotion. The new information by itself was not enough to eliminate the health hazard—tobacco use. Epidemiology and public health professionals began to focus their attention on efforts to change people's behavior, to help and encourage them to quit smoking or not to start, and to evaluate the effectiveness of different health education approaches to smoking cessation.

Research on smoking as well as other risk factors for cancer and cardiovascular disease (diet, exercise, and alcohol consumption, for example) helped catalyze a shift in epidemiology and public health to a concern with people's behavior. Research raised such questions as the physician's role in educating patients, the best way to inform the public about risks to health, and how to encourage life style changes. Slowly, over the thirty years since the Surgeon General's report, public policy has affected the labeling and advertising of cigarettes, smoking in public places, and the taxation of cigarettes. Epidemiology has moved beyond looking at the biological causes of disease to studying the interaction between medicine, public policy, health information, and behavioral changes. Thus, the investigation of smoking and lung cancer became linked with the story of smoking and heart disease and part of the greater effort to modify major risk factors for many illnesses in the general population.

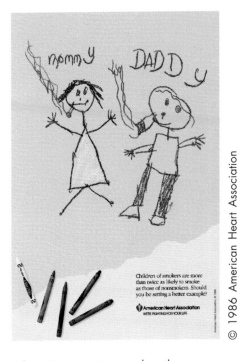

Advertising campaigns, such as the one by the American Heart Association that produced this poster, have informed the public about the dangers of smoking.

Other Causes of Cancer

EPIDEMIOLOGIC tools have been used to identify other causes of cancer and to point out new avenues of investigation. Epidemiologic research has been useful in pointing out the relationship between *in-utero* exposures and subsequent development of cancer, and of occupational exposures and sunlight as factors in the origin of various cancers.

Epidemiologists suggested that diet might also be a factor in explaining some cancers. Harold F. Dorn, William Haenszel, Abraham Lilienfeld, Irving Kessler, and others compared deaths from cancers in different geographical areas in efforts to discern patterns. Incidence of and mortality from different cancers vary from country to country, and this variation has suggested several hypotheses. One was that international variations in diet could explain international variations in some cancers. Plotting in-

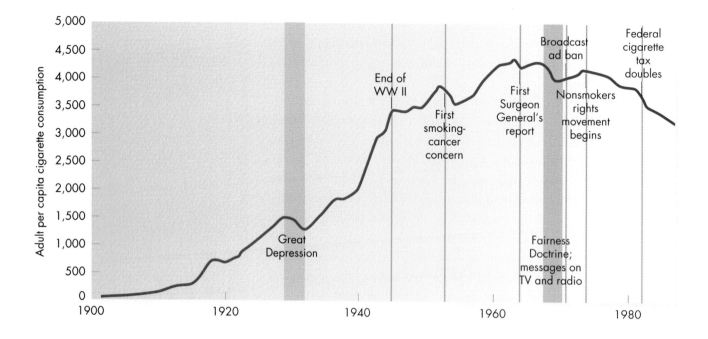

Research reports, changes in advertising, and cigarette taxes—all seem to have contributed to the downward trend in cigarette consumption.

cidence of cancer by national per capita dietary intake showed, for example, that daily meat consumption was associated with colon cancer in women, while daily fat intake was associated with uterine cancer. These studies have led to further exploration of the role of diet, particularly fat and meat consumption, in the development of colon and other cancers.

Geographic mapping of cancer incidence also provided clues to the understanding of skin cancer, but the relationship between sunlight exposure and skin cancer is complicated by the role of skin color in protecting the individual from sunlight. Dermatologists had noted the greater occurrence of skin cancer in parts of the body exposed to the sun; fair-skinned people, moreover, are at greater risk of developing skin cancer. Both sunlight and ultraviolet radiation were shown to cause skin cancer in rats and mice in the 1920s and 1930s, and by 1959 the carcinogenic portion of the spectrum was identified. Pigment in the skin protects against the harmful effects of sunlight by blocking ultraviolet radiation, and in the United States blacks have a much lower mortality from melanoma than do

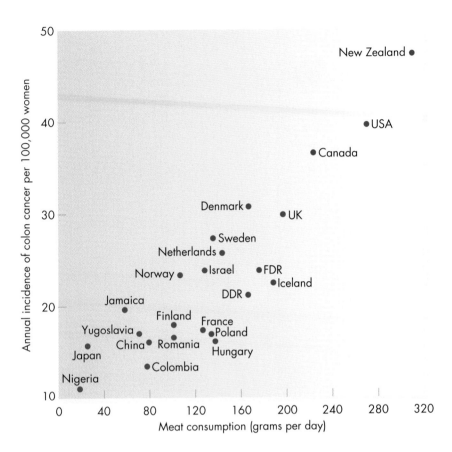

By correlating national statistics, epidemiologists are able to identify factors that may be associated with cancers; in this case, higher meat consumption appears to be correlated with an increased incidence of colon cancer in women. Such ecological studies are the beginnings of the epidemiologic approach to understanding the causes of cancer.

whites, even with a presumably similar exposure to sunlight. A genetic trait—skin color—protects against an environmental carcinogen—sunlight—to represent one example of the interaction between an individual's genetic makeup and the environment.

An Ironic Twist: A Bacterial Cause of Cancer

ALTHOUGH the story of cancer epidemiology revolves around the concept of multiple, noninfectious causes, a bacterial cause of one type of cancer, stomach cancer, has recently been suggested. In 1989, the name *Helicobacter pylori* was given to a newly discovered bacterium often found in the pyloris, an area between the stomach and the small intestine. The

This nineteenth-century drawing from a clinical textbook shows several forms of cancer, of which the middle two are skin cancer.

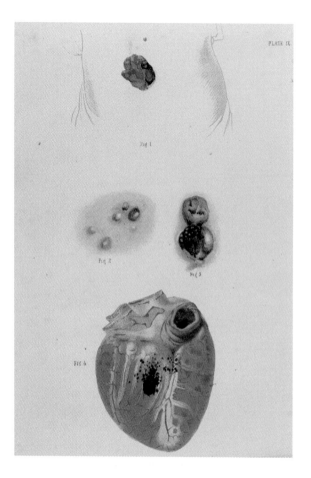

Australian physicians, J. Robin Warren and Barry J. Marshall, had investigated *H. pylori's* effects by following in the tradition of Goldberger and other medical scientists: they experimented on themselves. Barry Marshall drank a broth of active *H. pylori* bacteria; a week later he was nauseous, had stomach pains, and his breath was foul. A sample of his stomach contents during the second week revealed an active bacterial infection. Marshall and Warren suggested that the bacteria might be the cause of peptic ulcers, gastritis, or both. Since gastritis was thought to be associated with stomach cancer, even in their first paper Warren and Marshall were able to suggest that the bacteria play a role in that type of cancer.

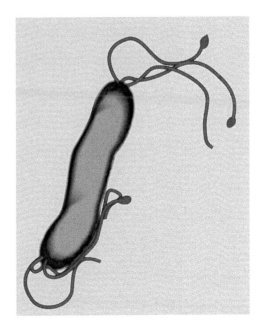

Helicobacter pylori, a bacterium first isolated in 1982, is strongly associated with ulcers, chronic gastritis, and stomach cancer.

The plausibility of a relationship between *H. pylori* and stomach cancer led researchers to compare the geographical distribution of the putative causal agent and the disease. Areas of the United States and of the world that show high prevalences of infection with *H. pylori* also showed high incidences of gastric carcinoma. This did not, by itself, prove a causal relationship between the two variables, but it is basic to the epidemiologic approach. It was a step in gathering the facts that, put together in a logical way, will form a cohesive argument for or against causality.

In 1991, shortly after the observation of geographical associations between *H. pylori* and stomach cancer, four case-control studies were published, quantifying and confirming that *H. pylori* is associated with stomach cancer. The studies used frozen blood samples or stored tissue slides to demonstrate *H. pylori* infection in gastric cancer patients at or before the time of diagnosis. About 60 percent of the patients had histories of infection. Having such a history multiplied the risk of developing stomach cancer: the odds ratio ranged from 1.6 to 17.7, suggesting a strong association between *H. pylori* infection and stomach cancer.

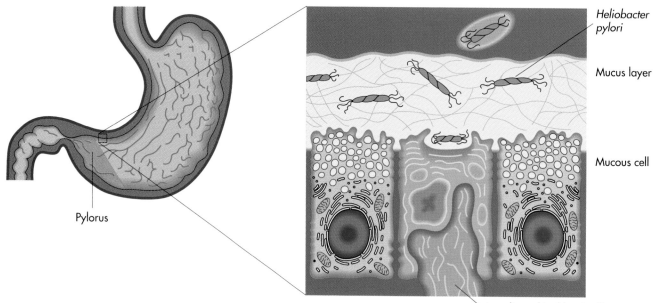

Pylorus

Heliobacter pylori

Mucus layer

Mucous cell

Invading white blood cell

Helicobacter pylori prefers the less acidic environment near the pylorus. Before *H. pylori* was discovered, it had been believed that no bacteria could survive the intensely acidic environment of the stomach. To protect itself from stomach acid, *H. pylori* lives in the mucus layer that lines the stomach, where the pH is neutral. Moreover, the bacteria produce a potent chemical that buffers its immediate environment so that it can survive for brief periods in the stomach itself. Cells from the immune system (leukocytes) attack cells to which the bacteria have attached themselves; it is in fact the activity of the immune system that creates the inflammation of an ulcer or gastritis.

One of these studies showed that the severity of *H. pylori* infection was correlated with the risk of gastric cancer—that is, patients with higher levels of antibody to *H. pylori* were most likely to develop stomach cancer. This finding of a dose relationship and the consistency of results across four studies further supported the hypothesis that the bacterium may cause stomach cancer. Prospective studies and efforts to decrease the incidence of stomach cancer by treating *H. pylori* infection would be the next steps in assessing the causal hypothesis.

A Biological Explanation for Epidemiologic Findings

ALTHOUGH epidemiology has contributed to our understanding of a variety of cancers and the exposures that cause them, the story of smoking and lung cancer illustrates particularly well the way that epidemiology can be used to identify a cause of disease (cigarette smoking) and a means of prevention (encouraging smoking cessation) even when the biology is not fully understood. In fact, epidemiologic evidence preceded biological understanding. Epidemiology can be a powerful science for this reason, but doubt is often cast on epidemiologic evidence because biological theories of disease are often not developed enough to explain epidemiologic findings.

Since the 1950s, the fields of molecular biology, genetics, immunology, and oncology have advanced greatly, providing us with an understanding of cancer biology and explanations for epidemiologic observations of the many causes associated with cancer.

The unregulated division and growth of cells that is cancer arises after a number of events occur:

- The cell loses its ability to repair mistakes in DNA synthesis (loses a so-called suppressor gene).
- The cell acquires the ability to promote unregulated growth (an inactive gene becomes inappropriately active, an active gene becomes excessively active, or a gene becomes active in an abnormal way).

A series of genetic changes must take place for cancer to result. In one proposed model for colon cancer, the full-blown disease develops only after tumor suppressor genes (*DCC* and *p53*) have been lost and growth-regulating genes *(ras)* activated. The mutation of one or two genes produces an adenoma, a group of irregular cells that is not yet malignant. There is no strong evidence that the mutations of the *ras*, *p53*, and *DCC* genes must happen in a particular order.

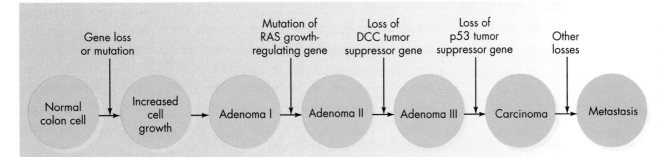

Exposure to radiation or chemicals can cause highly localized mutations or breakages in a strand of DNA or chromosome, and either type of damage can result in the loss of necessary functions or the gain of extra, undesired activities. That many exposures can cause these molecular changes, and that an array of cellular changes can lead to cancerous growth, explains the epidemiologic findings that many factors are associated with cancer.

Among the oldest reactions to the epidemiologic evidence about smoking and lung cancer were outcries such as "but my grandmother smoked a pack a day and lived to the age of ninety" or "my cousin never smoked, but died of lung cancer, anyway." We now know that individuals vary in their response to exposures to such carcinogens as ultraviolet radiation, x-rays, and tobacco smoke. Our cells and tissues have mechanisms that enable us to repair damage to DNA and to metabolize toxins; as individuals we vary in our success at coping with similar levels of exposure, and this variation can be a reflection of genetic differences in repair mechanisms.

In addition, it is now known that we carry varying susceptibility to individual types of cancer. A gene for colon cancer susceptibility and a gene for breast cancer susceptibility have been identified and located. Epidemiologic data collected by Mary-Claire King and her colleagues showed that women with breast cancer were more likely to have close relatives (sisters, daughters, or mothers) who had breast cancer than were women without breast cancer. This case-control study was used to gather evidence in support of the hypothesis that heredity is one determinant of the risk for breast cancer.

King then identified families in which more than three first-degree relatives had breast cancer (a mother and two daughters; three sisters; a grandmother, a mother, and a daughter). She eventually collected pedigrees of 23 families with 146 cases of breast cancer; blood samples taken from every family member were used for genetic analysis. These families would be most likely carry a gene for breast cancer. Blood samples provided DNA for analysis, and the researchers could begin lab work aimed at locating the gene for breast cancer. King and her group focused their studies on the long arm of the seventeenth chromosome because several genes related to normal breast development and possibly to breast cancer are found there. By studying the pattern of inheritance of genetic markers (linkage analysis), King was able to narrow the probable location of the gene for breast cancer susceptibility. Mary-Claire King and others continued their studies until in 1994 Mark H. Skolnick and his many colleagues announced their discovery of the precise location of the gene. Although its function remains uncertain, the gene could well turn out to be a tumor suppressor gene able to repair damaged DNA or to destroy cells with damaging mutations.

Whether or not they contain the gene for cancer, cells may not become cancerous until an exposure affects them. When a person carries a gene for breast cancer or colon cancer, all the cells in that organ have the gene and are one step further along the way toward cancer. Environmental exposures that cause additional mutations then accelerate the progression toward cancer.

As we are able to identify more of the genetic or chromosomal variations responsible for individual differences in risk or susceptibility, epidemiologists will be able to describe the distribution of these traits in the population. One example is variation in a molecule, p53. In 1993, *Science* magazine chose p53 as its "Molecule of the Year." p53 is a protein with a variety of functions related to the regulation of cell growth and division. It suppresses tumor growth and can trigger cell death in response to DNA damage (thereby preventing an abnormal cell from dividing). Epidemiologists, working with oncologists, cell biologists, and virologists, have documented more than 51 types of cancer that carry p53 mutations, and have found p53 mutations in half the people diagnosed with cancer. Moreover, they have found a variety of mutations that affect the conformation of the p53 molecule and affect its function. Each type of mutation produces a unique effect on the molecule; thus, it may be possible to link specific exposures to specific p53 mutations and, in turn, to specific cancers. For example, some mutations may be more likely to result from exposure to benzo(a)pyrene, a carcinogen in tobacco smoke, while others may be more likely to arise from exposure to aflatoxins, a

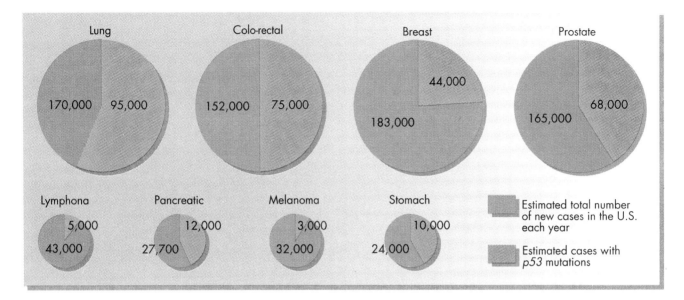

The beginnings of the molecular epidemiology of *p53* mutations: the estimated numbers of *p53* mutations in some common cancers in the United States. Mutations of the *p53* gene have been observed in nearly half of all cancers and in almost every type of cancer, although in some types they are less common than in others. Epidemiologists will have to work with oncologists, molecular biologists, and others to unravel the significance of these findings.

group of carcinogens associated with liver cancer. The pattern of mutations in the p53 molecule may tell us whether a cancer resulted from a specific environmental carcinogen.

Epidemiologic studies of p53 and its mutations will tell us the distribution of mutations in different populations exposed to different carcinogens and manifesting different cancers. When that information is combined with biological information about the molecule and its role in the cell, the result will be a more precise understanding of the relationship between exposure and disease, the risks associated with different exposures, and the mechanisms explaining the differences observed. Future epidemiologic studies about breast cancer will surely document the presence or absence of genes for breast cancer, as well as other genes and molecules thought to contribute to breast cancer susceptibility.

The epidemiologic approach produced information about cancer that had immediate health benefits well in advance of our biological knowledge. Epidemiology's encounter with cancer produced new methods and techniques, particularly the development of the case-control study and the use of the odds ratio, and it broadened our concepts of causality to account for the multiple pathways leading to cancer. The interaction of epidemiology and biology is somewhat like the game leapfrog: molecular and genetic advances now provide tools and direction for future epidemiologic investigations about the occurrence and distribution of cancer in the population.

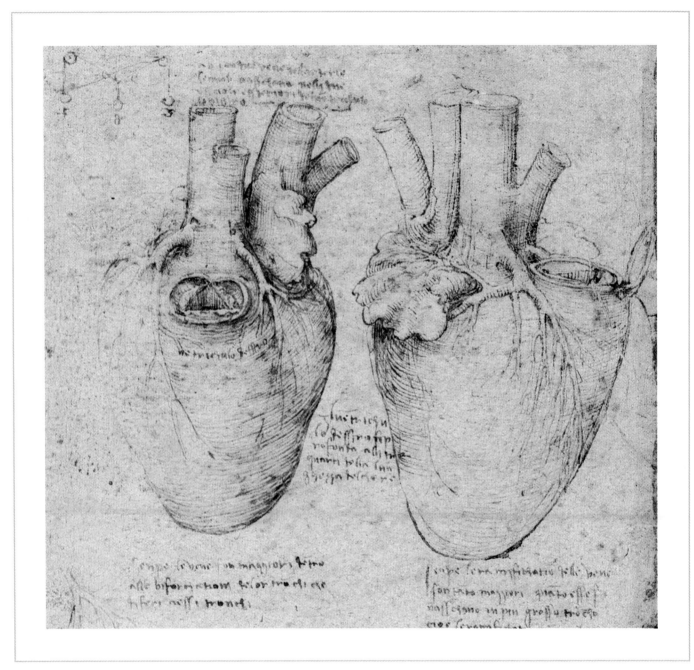

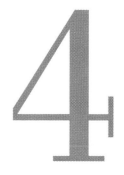

Heart Disease: Untangling the Risk Factors

ARTISTIC GRACE and intelligent observation combine in this drawing by Leonardo da Vinci, showing the distribution of arteries leading from the heart muscle. The factors that put these arteries at risk of blockage, and the heart at risk of an attack, have been objects of study for epidemiologists.

The beginning of the physician's secret: knowledge of the heart's movement and knowledge of the heart. There are vessels from it to every limb. As to this, when any physician, any surgeon, or any exorcist applies the hands or his fingers to the head, to the back of the head, to the hands, to the place of the stomach, to the arms or to the feet, then he examines the heart, because all his limbs possess its vessels, that is: the heart speaks out of the vessels of every limb.

So the Egyptians wrote in the Ebers papyrus of 1522 B.C. Diseases of the heart were recognized in ancient times, and Greco-Roman writings described sudden death and characteristics of the pulse. When the heart stopped, and a person's pulse ceased, life stopped. Although the heart's importance was clear, its function was not understood until the seventeenth century, when William Harvey discovered that the contractions of the heart propel blood out through the arteries and that the blood returns to the heart through the veins.

The heart is a muscle that pumps blood throughout our bodies, supplying our organs with nutrients and oxygen, and taking away carbon dioxide and other products of cell metabolism. The heart itself needs to be well nourished with blood that passes through arteries leading back into its tissues. When these arteries are blocked, oxygen supply to the heart muscle decreases, and the muscle is damaged or destroyed in a heart attack, more formally called a myocardial infarction. Veins leading to the heart, brain, or other organs can be suddenly blocked by circulating clots, or slowly constricted by the buildup of plaques (atherosclerosis) in the vessel linings. Such a buildup in the artery walls reduces the flow of blood and also increases the likelihood of a clot causing a blockage; a narrow artery is more readily blocked than a wide artery.

Although heart disease was recognized for centuries, it could be studied only after the development of tools to observe the heart and blood pressure. In 1819, René-Théophile-Hyacinthe Laennec published his work describing and interpreting the sounds heard through his invention,

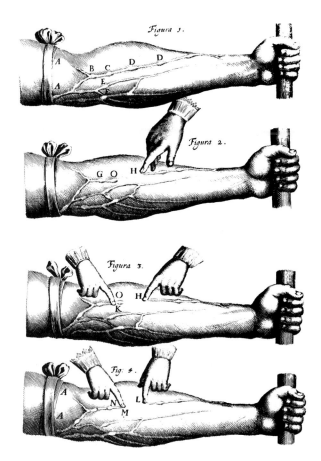

In this sketch, William Harvey illustrated that restricting the flow of blood in an artery leading away from the heart results in a corresponding decrease in blood flow in the vein leading back to the heart. In effect, Harvey has demonstrated the circulation of blood from heart to limbs, head, and organs and back to the heart again.

the stethoscope. Although Laennec applied the stethoscope to the diagnosis and study of respiratory disease, the instrument opened the way for study of the heart's sounds and their relation to disease. Similarly, the development between 1896 and 1905 of a clinically useful sphygmomanometer allowed the study of blood pressure and its relation to disease. Until then, cardiovascular disease could be recognized only when a person experienced chest pain or died of a stroke or heart attack. Tools for listening to the heart and observing blood pressure enabled scientists to begin to observe cardiovascular function, collect data, and form hypotheses about disease.

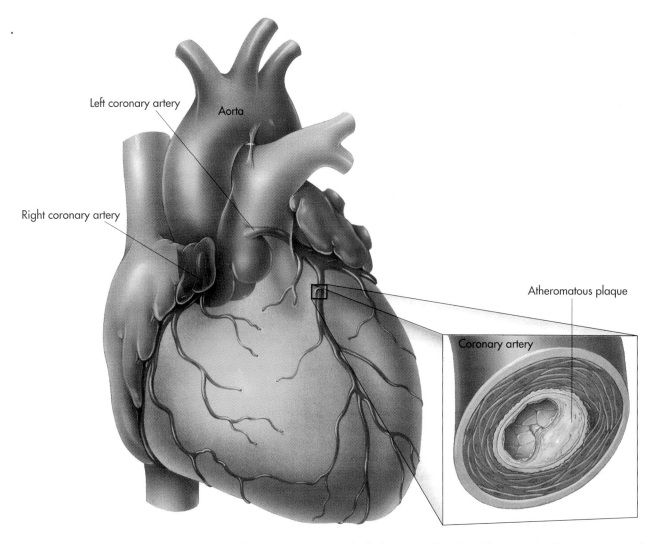

Left coronary artery

Aorta

Right coronary artery

Atheromatous plaque

Coronary artery

Coronary arteries supply the heart muscle with its blood supply. The cross section of an artery shows the narrowing caused by the buildup of artherosclerotic plaque. When the coronary arteries become occluded, they can easily be blocked by clots, and blood supply to the heart muscle is restricted.

Cardiology texts of the early twentieth century considered most heart disease to be the consequence of syphilis and rheumatic fever, and perhaps this impression accurately reflected the nineteenth-and early-twentieth-century reality that infectious diseases caused much of the heart disease of the time. Heart disease was not recognized as a problem in its own right.

As infectious diseases waned in importance, and as increasing proportions of the population lived longer, coronary heart disease became recognized as a disease with its own etiology. In 1910, heart disease became the leading cause of death in the United States and, except for the years from 1918 to 1920 when influenza was pandemic, it has remained so to the present. The percentage of deaths attributable to heart disease peaked in 1968 at 35 percent, up from 8 percent in 1900 and 27 percent in 1950. The absolute number of deaths from the disease peaked in 1963, when an estimated 541,000 people died from the effects of heart disease.

The elimination of many infectious causes of mortality allowed more people to live longer and die of other causes, notably cancer and cardiovascular diseases, but longer life spans did not explain all of the increase in heart disease, just as they did not for cancer. Cigarette smoking was a new habit characterizing modern twentieth-century life and explained a substantial proportion of the rise in lung cancer and coronary heart disease alike, but other behaviors also contributed to the increased risk of heart disease.

Epidemiology's attention to cardiovascular disease research led to a decline in mortality from the disease and to a more complete understanding of the factors contributing to it. As with cancer epidemiology, cardiovascular epidemiologists applied their techniques to a new area of medicine, and brought new concepts and methods to their field, including the risk factor, multiple regression analytic methods for epidemiologic data, and the maturation of the randomized clinical trial. Thus the story of cardiovascular epidemiology encompasses some of the greatest advances in the history of the discipline.

The Framingham Heart Study and Multiple Risks

CRUCIAL in defining the issues for epidemiological investigation of heart disease has been the Framingham Heart Study, often cited as a prototype of a prospective cohort study, in which a group, or cohort, is described and then studied over time to document changes in its members' health. The Framingham study involved a collaboration between the Massachusetts Department of Health, Harvard Medical School, and the U.S. Public Health Service. During 1948 and 1949, a cohort of 5,209 people aged 30 to 59 and free of cardiovascular disease was enrolled. They were then reexamined every two years. This group is still under observation, but reports have been released at intervals, beginning in 1961.

The accumulated data suggested that more than one factor could be associated with the probability of experiencing a myocardial infarction and of dying from cardiovascular disease. It was not known whether these factors were causes of heart disease, but they were statistically and temporally associated with the risk of heart disease. The Framingham study's report of 1961 coined the phrase "risk factors" to describe such associations. Initial data showed that the risk of heart disease was greater in males than females, and that it increased with age, blood pressure, and the amount of cholesterol in the blood (serum cholesterol).

Over the years the Framingham Study—confined to the residents of the town of Framingham, Massachusetts—has expanded beyond the original cohort of middle-aged men to include even children.

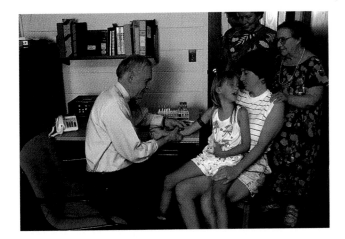

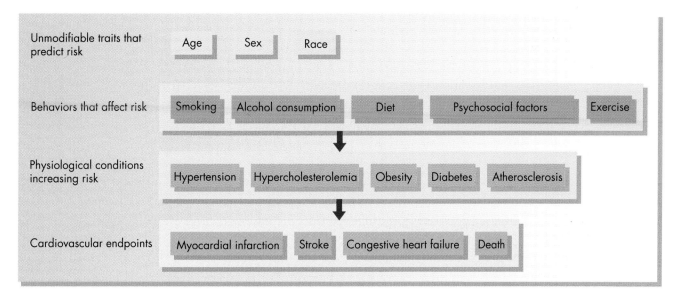

Unmodifiable traits that predict risk	Age	Sex	Race		
Behaviors that affect risk	Smoking	Alcohol consumption	Diet	Psychosocial factors	Exercise
Physiological conditions increasing risk	Hypertension	Hypercholesterolemia	Obesity	Diabetes	Atherosclerosis
Cardiovascular endpoints	Myocardial infarction	Stroke	Congestive heart failure	Death	

From the first analysis of the Framingham data, it was necessary to consider the effect of each variable in the context of other risk factors for heart disease. Heart disease was clearly different from infectious diseases, where a single pathogen caused a single disease—and different even from lung cancer, for which cigarette smoking was the main risk factor. A number of elements appeared to independently increase the risk of heart disease, but in order to describe their effects, statistical methods that could account for the effect of more than one independent variable were needed. Stratified analysis (separating groups into smaller groups of different combinations of risk factors) was employed in the first decades of the Framingham study. For example, observations were grouped or cross-tabulated by smoking status, glucose intolerance, ECG (electrocardiogram) findings, and cholesterol levels, and then compared within each group with respect to the effect of blood pressure on the probability of coronary heart disease. Groups with higher blood pressures showed higher probabilities of coronary heart disease, whatever the coexisting factors.

By the 1970s, computers had made possible the more widespread use of multiple regression and related statistical techniques that helped describe the joint effects of several risk factors on the probability of devel-

Demographic characteristics, behavioral practices, physiological characteristics all affect our risk of cardiovascular disease.

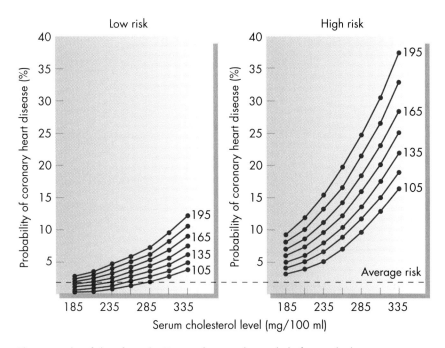

These graphs of data from the Framingham study, made before multiple regression statistical models came into wide use, use a visual format to present the influence of multiple risk factors on coronary heart disease. The graphs compare two groups of men: the high-risk group were smokers, with glucose intolerance and ECG abnormalities, and the low-risk group were nonsmokers, without glucose intolerance or ECG abnormalities. Within each group patients are stratified by blood pressure levels (each curved line represents a blood pressure level). Higher blood pressure levels are consistently associated with higher risks of coronary heart disease. For each blood pressure level, risk of heart disease increases with serum cholesterol measures, demonstrating that higher cholesterol levels increase the risk of heart disease independent of blood pressure, and for both the low-risk and high-risk groups.

oping heart disease. Multiple regression techniques are mathematical models (equations) that allow us to look at more than two variables at a time. They provide estimates of the amount of change caused in one variable when another variable is changed by a given unit, *and* other variables are also in the model. For example, the techniques can be used to

Changes in the Recognition and Treatment of Hypertension

	National Health Survey (1960–2)	National Community Evaluation Clinic (1973–5)	Chicago (1977)
Number of people examined	6,672	1,049,225	177,692
Hypertensives (blood pressure > 160/95)	18%	22%	8%
Hypertensives unaware of diagnosis	58%	28%	7%
Hypertensives being treated	21%	62%	93%
Hypertensives under control	16%	45%	73%

show how changes in serum cholesterol level alter the risk of heart disease after mathematically adjusting for levels of other variables such as blood pressure, smoking, diabetes, and so on.

Hypertension (high blood pressure) showed up early in the Framingham study as having a consistent association with heart disease. Within subgroups of smokers or nonsmokers, people with high cholesterol or people with low cholesterol, and so on, increases in blood pressure were directly correlated with increases in heart disease. This consistent relationship may reflect the increased burden on the heart placed by high blood pressure as greater effort is needed to push the blood through the arteries.

The awareness of hypertension's adverse effects on health led to more aggressive screening, identification, and treatment of high blood pressure, as well as greater comprehension of such issues as patient education and factors that influence adherence to treatment. The table above shows substantial increases over time in the number of people aware of their blood pressure, those being treated for hypertension, and those whose hypertension was under control. The National Health Survey of 1960–2 showed that 58 percent of hypertensives were unaware of their hypertension; in 1977 the Chicago survey found this number dropped to 7 percent. These same surveys showed an increase in the number of hypertensives who were being treated. Current medical practice is to monitor blood pressure,

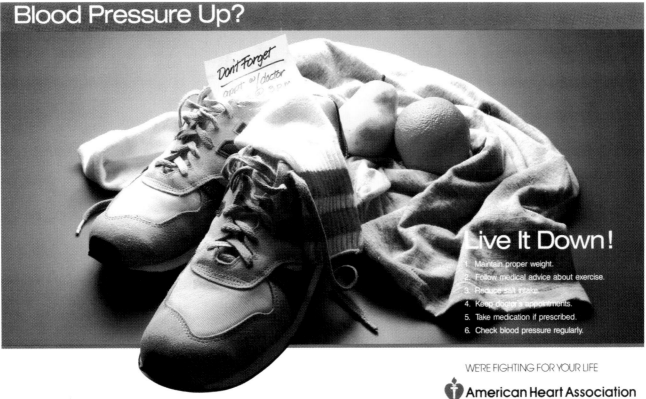

Blood Pressure Up?

Don't Forget
appt w/ doctor
@ 3 P.M.

Live It Down!

1. Maintain proper weight.
2. Follow medical advice about exercise.
3. Reduce salt intake.
4. Keep doctor's appointments.
5. Take medication if prescribed.
6. Check blood pressure regularly.

WE'RE FIGHTING FOR YOUR LIFE
American Heart Association

Information gathered by epidemiologists contributes to public health efforts to lower the incidence of heart disease. This poster suggests ways that people can modify their risk of heart disease, particularly by controlling their blood pressure.

encourage patients to be aware of their blood pressure, and treat hypertension long before it manifests itself in the other clinical conditions that may follow when high blood pressure is left uncontrolled.

The Risk Factor Cholesterol

THE connection between cholesterol and atherosclerosis has been known since early in the century, when, between 1908 and 1912, it was demonstrated in animals by A. Ignatowski, N. N. Anitschkow, and their colleagues. These Russian scientists produced atherosclerosis in rabbits by feeding the animals a diet high in cholesterol, which is one of the molecules, known as lipids, that constitute fatty foods like butter and oil. Their experimental evidence was initially dismissed, however, as irrelevant to health in humans; cholesterol was not a normal part of a rabbit's diet, and that supposedly explained why rabbits became sick from high-cholesterol diets. Nonetheless, researchers began to explore the associations between diet, serum cholesterol levels, and atherosclerosis. By the 1930s, geographical comparisons showed that countries with high-fat diets (like the United States) had high levels of atherosclerotic disease. Moreover, people who moved from countries with low-fat diets and low levels of heart disease (like Japan) to areas of high-fat diets (the United States) acquired the higher risk of heart disease. Indeed, the more years the immigrants had resided in their adopted country, the greater the difference between their chances of acquiring heart disease and their former compatriot's chances. The Framingham study confirmed the conclusion already suggested by the accumulated evidence. Cholesterol levels were indeed associated with heart disease, and as early as 1961 the American Heart Association suggested that decreased intake of cholesterol could alter blood cholesterol levels and lower the risk of atherosclerotic disease.

In the years since, study after study has added to the evidence that high cholesterol is a cause of heart disease. The studies include at least 12 analyses of data collected by the Food and Agriculture Organization along with the World Health Organization, analyses of 31,000 autopsies from 15 countries, field studies, migration studies, and comparisons of populations within countries. A review published in 1981 cited data from 65 cohorts in 23 countries, all using multivariate analyses. Some studies attained enormous sample sizes, like the Multiple Risk Factor Intervention Trial (MRFIT), which screened 361,662 men aged 35 to 57. In the MRFIT study, men from 18 U.S. cities were examined between 1973 and 1975 and their mortality monitored for 16 years. The large numbers allowed the investigators to make comparisons between more than one subgroup and to make precise estimates of effect by using multiple regression analyses. An increase in total cholesterol from 190 to 230 milligrams per deciliter (mg/dl) of blood appeared to increase the risk of death from coronary heart disease by 30 percent, after controlling for the independent effects of blood pressure, smoking, diabetes, race, income, and age.

In the early 1960s, the evidence for a causal relationship between cholesterol and heart disease was strong enough for epidemiologists to recommend that people reduce their cholesterol levels as a means of lowering their risk of heart disease. But epidemiologists hadn't yet shown that the recommended course of action actually worked—that eating less fat could help prevent coronary illness. While research had demonstrated that high cholesterol could cause heart disease, it was necessary next to establish that a reduction in cholesterol levels could reduce one's risk of heart disease. It was also necessary to demonstrate that individuals could reduce their serum cholesterol levels. The body produces some of its own cholesterol, and stores cholesterol as well; perhaps the body would compensate for lower cholesterol intake and maintain serum cholesterol levels. In that case, reducing cholesterol in the diet would not necessarily reduce cholesterol in the blood. Epidemiologists needed to conduct formal studies of the impact of dietary intake on cholesterol levels.

The first step in such a study is to teach individuals to change their diets. Then one must document that they have indeed changed their diets, describe their health over several years, and compare their diet, cholesterol levels, and the incidence of coronary heart disease to a similar group of people who did not begin a special program to change their cholesterol intake.

Changes in diet are appealing ways to fight disease because they may be safe, inexpensive, and accessible to most of the population. But evaluating the efficacy of a change in diet is difficult because it takes a long time to teach people to alter what they eat. Indeed, just describing dietary changes may become quite involved. One problem is that most of us eat varied diets that change from weekday to weekend, from season to season, and with special occasions. Thus, it is more useful to collect information over several days than for a single day. A second problem is that although we may wish to study a substance like cholesterol, people do not eat pure cholesterol—they eat foods that may contain cholesterol. It is difficult for people to estimate how much they ate of Aunt Muriel's stuffed cabbage,

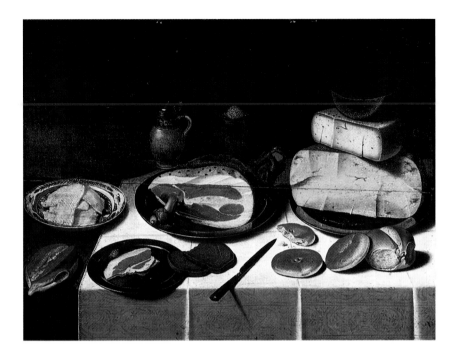

High-fat foods such as beef, pork, cheese, eggs, and cream have long been staples of many European cuisines, as illustrated by this seventeenth-century painting, and they are abundant in American cooking as well. People raised on such diets may find it difficult to alter their eating habits and lower their fat intake.

how much chopped meat was in the portion, and how fatty Aunt Muriel's meat was. People may accurately recall the amount of butter they spread on toast each morning, but do they also remember the two crackers with dip that they had when dropping by an office party? or that they ate the last third of their child's ice cream cone?

A further problem is that to describe dietary intake people need to keep careful records of the amounts and types of food eaten—and such record keeping often causes people to change their eating habits (indeed, weight-loss programs may use diaries as a step in helping people control their eating). Even when one assigns people to groups randomly, one group receiving dietary instruction and modifying their diets and another group not receiving any instruction, researchers cannot prevent the members of the uninstructed group from changing their diets also. Members of the uninstructed group may be convinced by information received elsewhere to reduce their consumption of fatty foods, and then the two groups may become similar in their intake of cholesterol.

Because of the difficulties posed by diet studies, investigators turned to another, more rigorous method of establishing the causal relationship between serum cholesterol and heart disease. They undertook to describe accurately and in great detail the effect of cholesterol-lowering drugs on serum cholesterol and heart disease.

The Randomized Controlled Clinical Trial

CHOLESTEROL levels can be lowered not only by a change in diet, but also by drugs such as cholestyramine. Such drugs are, of course, thoroughly tested before they go on the market, and the testing method is the most scientifically rigorous type of study available to the epidemiologist—the randomized, controlled clinical trial. After demonstrating the safety and efficacy of the treatment, epidemiologists carry out larger, more extensive clinical trials to describe the effects of treatment on health—in the case of cholestyramine, that reducing serum cholesterol levels can lead to a reduction in heart disease.

Randomized controlled clinical trials have several advantages over cohort studies, whether "historical" or prospective. In cohort studies, people self-select into study groups by various criteria: people choose to smoke or not to smoke, workers' abilities and personalities determine their job placements and, in turn, some of their exposures. In designing such observational studies, the researcher needs to think through the variables that determine selection into groups and to control for such variables in design or analysis. Since exposure is not controlled by the researcher, these designs are particularly prone to confounding: an unequal distribution of extraneous factors may explain the outcome of such studies.

The randomized controlled clinical trial allows the investigator to (1) randomly allocate patients to study groups and (2) assign groups to treatments or placebos. When patients are randomly allocated to groups, patient characteristics should be distributed randomly between the two groups. The study groups should end up resembling each other in age, sex, height, weight, smoking patterns, economic status, occupations, diet, other medical conditions, and any other variable that could affect the study outcome. The two (or more) groups then differ only with respect to the experimental treatment. The investigator assigns one group to one type of drug, diet, therapy, procedure, or other treatment, and other groups to alternative treatments or to no treatment. If the study groups are similar at the start of the trial, then differences observed at the completion of the trial can be attributed to the treatments.

Ideally, all treatment groups receive a form of treatment; even the group that receives no treatment receives a "placebo" that is indistinguishable from the experimental treatment but has no effect. When the health care provider and patient are unaware of their treatment status ("blinded"), the patient's or researcher's ideas about the treatment cannot affect the way outcomes are perceived or recorded.

One such randomized, controlled clinical trial was the Lipid Research Clinics Coronary Primary Prevention Trial, which tested the effectiveness of the cholesterol-lowering drug cholestyramine in reducing coronary heart disease. This study was intended to evaluate not just total

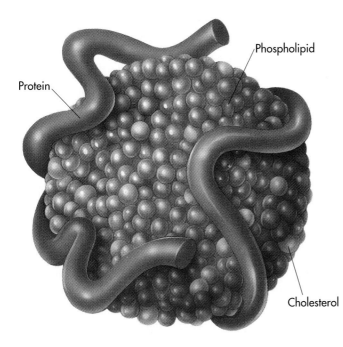

Protein

Phospholipid

Cholesterol

Two-thirds of the cholesterol in the blood is carried by low-density lipoproteins (LDLs). An LDL particle consists of about 2,000 molecules of cholesterol, 1,000 molecules of phospholipid, and a large protein that winds around the surface.

cholesterol but one particular type of cholesterol. Like all lipids, cholesterol does not travel through the blood as individual molecules; rather several thousand molecules are bound together with a protein to form a so-called lipoprotein. One type of cholesterol-containing lipoprotein—called low-density lipoprotein, or LDL—is especially likely to remain in the blood for several days and is thus especially likely to contribute to heart disease. For this reason, the researchers were careful to measure the amount of LDL-cholesterol in the blood.

Twelve clinics in the United States and Canada participated, screening 480,000 men aged 35 to 59 between July 1973 and July 1976. Men were eligible for the study if their cholesterol was 265 mg/dl or greater

The steps in the Lipid Research Clinics Primary Prevention Trial, a randomized, controlled clinical trial. In such a trial a target population is defined, eligibility criteria are established, and patients are allocated to one of two (or more) groups —the treatment group or the placebo group. Each group is followed for a set amount of time, and observed for the occurrence of disease—in this study, coronary heart disease.

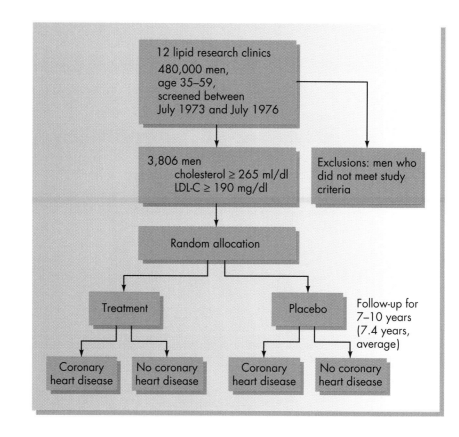

and their LDL-cholesterol in particular was 190 mg/dl or greater. During four successive screening visits, men were dropped from the study if their LDL-cholesterol levels fell below 175 mg/dl. Their removal eliminated from the group men who had borderline levels of LDL-cholesterol—men whose LDL fluctuated around the cutoff level of 190 mg/dl. At the fifth clinic visit, participants (having given informed consent to randomization) were randomly allocated to one of two groups: treatment or placebo. The caregivers and patients were "blind" to treatment status; all participants received pills (the treatment group got active medication, while the placebo group took inactive pills) and were cared for as if the pills were active.

The patients continued to visit the clinics for 7 to 10 years (7.4 years on average). Over this period, the cholestyramine group experienced 155 myocardial infarctions, both fatal and nonfatal, compared to 187 in the placebo group. Plotting the cumulative incidence over time, one can see that the cholestyramine group had fewer heart attacks in total, and that its members spent longer periods of time free of heart disease. Total cholesterol reductions were greater in the treatment group than in the placebo group. Moreover, the reduction in cholesterol showed a dose response: patients with greater adherence to the treatment (as measured by pill packet refills) showed greater decreases in total cholesterol and LDL-cholesterol. There was a consistent relationship between cholestyramine use, the lowering of total and LDL-cholesterol levels, and the reduction of coronary heart disease.

Randomized controlled clinical trials are expensive and time consuming. They involve the manipulation (rather than observation only) of humans, and are thus limited by ethical, legal, and practical constraints. A clinical trial must be stopped early if a treatment is found to be dangerous or clearly advantageous; it is not ethical to allow people to be harmed or deprived of an effective treatment. Patients must knowledgeably and freely give their consent to participate; participation in the trial cannot affect the patient's access to other aspects of their medical care; and patients need to be fully informed about risks and benefits associated with treatments or placebos. Finally, some forms of behavior are not amenable to experimental manipulation: new mothers cannot be assigned to breast

After the second year of the study, differences in the incidence of heart disease become apparent. The placebo group had higher levels of disease, and the differences between the placebo group and the treatment group grew wider with the passing of time.

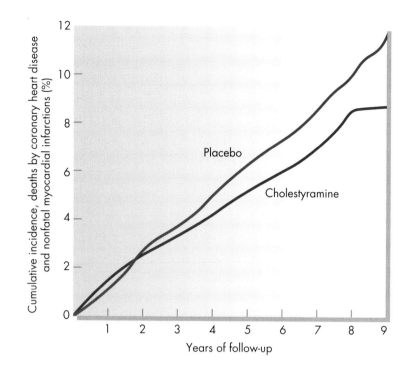

feed or bottle feed their infants to evaluate the effect of feeding practices on infant health, and couples may not readily agree to be assigned to different types of contraceptives in order to measure contraceptive efficacy.

The Lipids Research Clinics' randomized controlled clinical trial demonstrated that cholesterol-lowering drugs reduced serum cholesterol levels and the risk of coronary heart disease. The outcome of a randomized controlled clinical trial is the final piece of evidence needed in establishing causality. Epidemiologists, physicians, and public health workers had urged the public to reduce serum cholesterol before clinical trials had provided their results. The results of the trials accelerated the efforts to lower serum cholesterol and inspired many of the measures—such as the proper labeling of food fat content, the lowering of the fat content of school lunches, and the development of low-fat food products—that have been changing the public's attitude toward dietary fat.

The LDL Receptor

EPIDEMIOLOGISTS were not the only scientists interested in cholesterol. Biomedical researchers began to investigate how the body metabolizes the lipid molecules in fatty foods like butter and oils. In spite of their role in causing occluded arteries, lipids like cholesterol are necessary components of hormones and cell membranes and also serve as storehouses of energy. The body has mechanisms for maintaining and regulating the supply of lipids in the blood, but we may overburden these mechanisms by consuming too much fat or we may inherit genetic traits that limit our ability to regulate serum cholesterol. Biomedical research helped describe the body's mechanisms for using lipids and controlling the amounts that enter cells, as well as genetic defects leading to inadequate control of such physiological mechanisms. Michael Brown and Joseph Goldstein received the Nobel Prize for medicine in 1985 specifically for their work describing the regulation of LDL-cholesterol.

Certain individuals have a genetic predisposition to high serum cholesterol, a condition called hypercholesterolemia. Brown and Goldstein examined the genetic defects in patients who had the abnormally high cholesterol levels of hypercholesterolemia and who came from families where that condition was common. Hypercholesterolemia—serum cholesterol of 300 to 600 mg/dl, and LDL-cholesterol greater than 200 mg/dl—occurs in one in 500 people and one in twenty myocardial infarction patients younger than 60. Brown and Goldstein found that the gene for hypercholesterolemia, which has been mapped to chromosome 19, affects the function of particular proteins, called LDL receptors, on cell membranes. The function of the LDL receptor is to bind to the protein on the LDL-cholesterol lipoprotein so that the lipoprotein molecule can leave the bloodstream and enter the cell.

We now know of more than 35 mutations, all of that single gene, affecting the LDL receptor. Some of these mutations cause a cell to synthesize a receptor that is defective in binding LDL. Cells with other mutations may fail to transport the receptor to the cell surface or to locate the receptor correctly on the cell membrane or even to synthesize the recep-

Receptors in the cell membrane determine whether lipoproteins are bound and brought into the cell. Once inside the cell, the lipoprotein is broken down into its component amino acids and cholesterol molecules. If a high level of cholesterol enters, the cell slows its synthesis of both receptors and cholesterol.

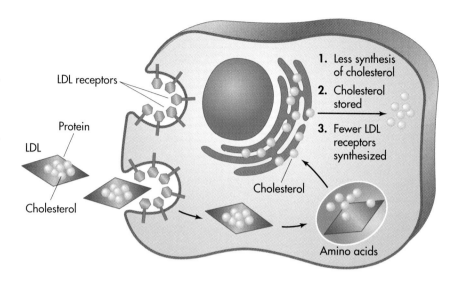

tor at all. In all these cases, cells are less able to bind LDL and incorporate cholesterol.

Their work on genetic variation in LDL regulation gave Brown and Goldstein insight into the normal regulation of LDL-cholesterol. The LDL receptors allow the cell to respond appropriately to variations in circulating LDL-cholesterol. When more LDL binds to a cell's receptors than the cell can process, it reduces its own synthesis of cholesterol and transforms more into a form suitable for storage. Most significantly for the course of heart disease, however, the cell stops synthesizing cell receptors at its usual rate. Whether the cause is a genetic mutation or over consumption of fat, when cells have a reduced number of LDL receptors available, LDL-cholesterol is left in the blood, where it can clog arteries and lead to heart attack.

Physical Activity and Cardiovascular Disease

EARLY cross-sectional studies showed an association between physical activity and heart disease. Conductors on London's double-decker buses experienced half the incidence of myocardial infarction observed in bus drivers. Postmen showed less heart disease than did otherwise similar but sedentary government employees. Although the physical activity associated with London fare collection (walking up and down the bus and climbing stairs to collect fares) or mail delivery might explain the lower level of heart disease, alternative explanations were also possible. Perhaps healthier, more vigorous people chose more active jobs and continued to be more healthy. Furthermore, people who developed illnesses or conditions that prevented physical activity might have transferred out of their demanding jobs, leaving an especially healthy group of people as bus conductors or mailmen. Finally, bus conductors and mailmen use their hands at work and may be less likely to smoke cigarettes on the job.

Prospective studies were necessary to describe the relationship between physical activity and heart disease. As people became involved in more sedentary occupations, physical activity became confined to leisure hours. Perhaps the amount and type of leisure physical activity affected an individual's risk of heart disease. A ten-year follow-up of 16,882 British male executive-grade civil servants showed that only vigorous activity (activities such as swimming, tennis, running, bicycling, and dancing that involve energy expenditures of 7.5 calories per minute or more) seemed to lower the incidence of coronary heart disease. An additional ten years of follow-up of 9,375 members of the cohort who were free of coronary heart disease found that high amounts of vigorous aerobic exercise seemed to protect against heart disease, but total energy expenditure did not. Physical exercise may directly benefit the heart and circulation, but it may also have a positive effect on weight, serum lipids, glucose metabolism, and blood pressure.

No one has successfully conducted a randomized controlled clinical trial assigning people to exercise regimens. In theory, one could assign people to different levels of exercise, perhaps by paying them to engage in different types of activity over a several-year period. In practice, the numbers of people needed, the inability to blind people to their "treatment" (exercise), and the problem of keeping people consistently within particular activity guidelines present problems difficult to overcome.

Without the option of a randomized trial, researchers have relied on observational studies to untangle the effects of physical activity on heart disease. Meta-analysis (the pooling of data from several studies) offers greater precision when there are many similar studies of a single research question. Jesse Berlin and Graham Colditz pooled results from 17 studies comparing workers in different occupations and 22 studies that looked at overall activity regardless of occupation. The studies compared three different levels of physical activity and several endpoints (death, myocardial infarction, angina pectoris, and so on). Individual studies may suffer from flaws such as small sample sizes, small contrasts in levels of physical activity, and equivocal findings that make firm conclusions difficult to draw. By pooling the data from many studies, Berlin and Colditz were able to conclude that lack of physical activity does indeed increase the risk of coronary heart disease. Exercise appears to help prevent heart attacks, but the data did not indicate that exercise reduces the severity of a heart attack should one occur.

While physical activity may protect a person from heart disease generally, incidents of sudden death during exercise have discouraged some from exercising (particularly older people or those with heart disease). People may experience heart attacks during exercise, as well as during sleep, reading, watching television, and other activities. But is the incidence of sudden death during exercise greater than would be expected on the basis of chance alone? Is it dangerous to engage in vigorous physical activity?

More than twenty studies have looked at the risk of sudden death during exercise. One study by David Siscovick and colleagues at the University of Washington examined both the overall protective effect of exercise and the risk of sudden death during exercise, given different habitual levels of exercise. Categorizing people according to the time spent each week in high-intensity physical activity, Siscovick showed a dose-response gradient: people who spent more time in high-intensity activity showed a greater overall protection from sudden death. When he compared the probability of dying during exercise to that during the rest of the day, he found an increased risk for all three exercising categories. Those who exercised least had the greatest increase in risk during exer-

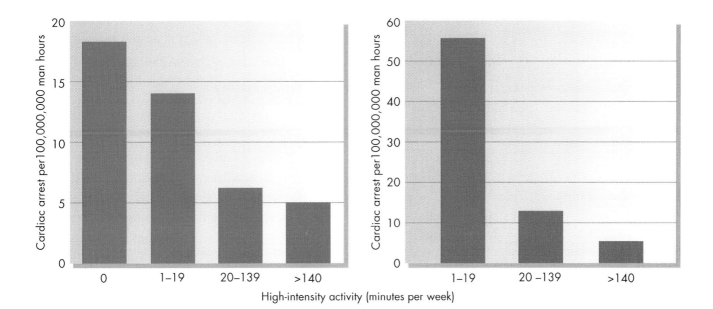

High-intensity activity (minutes per week)

cise (their risk during exercise was 50 times greater than during other time periods), while those who exercised most frequently showed a lower but definite increase in transient risk during exercise. Despite the increase during exercise, the overall risk was lowest in the group that exercised most.

Current medical practice encourages exercise in many patients with known heart disease, as well as the general population. Exercise can help people cope with stress, lose weight, improve their sense of well-being, reduce their risk of heart disease, and improve their health after heart disease is manifest. Research continues to address the many types of physical activity and its many effects, both immediate and long-term.

The overall risk of heart disease declines with increasing levels of high-intensity physical activity (left), although there is a transient increase in risk during exercise, which, for people with habitually low levels of high-intensity physical activity, is more than 50 times higher than their risk during other activities (right). Such findings are confusing for people who wish to know whether exercise is good from them or not.

Psychosocial Risk Factors

LEGEND, literature, and folk wisdom conceive of the heart as more than a muscle or mechanical pump, connecting it in some way to our emotions, personalities, and yearnings. Can emotions aggravate a heart condition?

Do certain personalities experience a greater risk of heart disease? Can tragic events cause a heart to "break" and lead to death? The metaphors of the heart are part of our culture, and scientists may consciously or unconsciously draw on such metaphors, or suggest hypotheses that resonate with cultural beliefs. Theories about the relationship between psychosocial factors and heart disease are at the same time appealing and seemingly unscientific.

Epidemiologists have taken a scientific approach to this body of hypotheses. Epidemiologic methods have been used to measure the effect of social class, job stress, social networks, life events, and personality on an individual's risk of heart disease. Such research depends on clear definitions of concepts like social class or stress, as well as on objective ways of measuring such factors. Defining and measuring a concept like stress can be difficult, however. Stress has been measured, for example, by asking people whether they have recently experienced events such as a death in the family, the loss of a job, a move to a new job, or a move to a new home. Yet an event such as the loss of a job may have different meanings to a fifty-five-year-old man after twenty years of employment at the same company than to someone who has changed jobs many times. Moreover, when measuring only such "acute" events, the researcher neglects to measure long-term sources of stress such as chronic unemployment, the responsibility for caring for an elderly dependent, a bad marriage, or a job with an excessive workload.

Various work characteristics have been associated with coronary heart disease, including working overtime, lack of authority over decisions, social isolation at work, job strain, and shift work. Sometimes the findings are difficult to interpret. The combination of high demands and low decision latitude, for example, is more of a predictor in blue-collar men than in white-collar men, and a modest level of overtime work was associated with stimulating work for men, but not for women.

A high number of social contacts in and out of work seems to increase one's chances of survival following a myocardial infarction. Perhaps social support helps a person take better care of him- or herself. Bereavement, migration, retirement, and other life events can be associated with heart disease, as can other significant life changes.

In the 1950s two California physicians, Meyer Friedman and Ray H. Rosenman, suggested that a certain personality type may be more likely to develop heart disease—the "Type A" person, who is angry, impatient, competitive and feels pressured about time. Research groups took this concept in several different directions, some defining Type A behavior as a response provoked by specific situations, others defining it as a stable trait. Type A behavior was not predictive of cardiovascular disease in the MRFIT study, but one component of Type A behavior, hostility, was.

It is plausible that psychosocial factors affect the risk of heart disease through both behavioral and physiological pathways. Perhaps psychosocial factors influence the release of hormones and these in turn have an effect on heart disease.

Research on psychosocial issues has helped to separate subjective impressions from scientific observation and show that a person's community and social environment can influence his or her health. The problem is that it may be impossible to put this knowledge to work preventing heart disease. People who are under stress, or lack social support, or have high levels or job dissatisfaction cannot usually change their environments or behaviors to lower their risk of heart disease. Some health care organizations have begun including wellness workshops addressing stress management, a worthy goal in itself, but it is not clear that such workshops reduce heart disease.

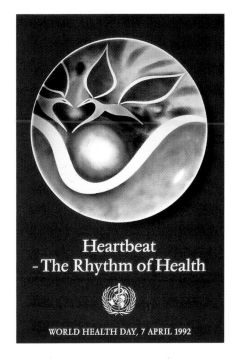

Heartbeat
- The Rhythm of Health

WORLD HEALTH DAY, 7 APRIL 1992

Heart disease was once primarily a concern of Western, industrialized nations. As this poster from the World Health Organization suggests, heart disease has become a global health concern as more and more of the world consumes a Westernized diet, exchanges physical work for desk jobs, and takes up cigarette smoking.

An Epidemiological Victory

At the beginning of this chapter we described the rise in incidence of heart disease and its associated mortality that began at the turn of the century, when heart disease first was recognized as the leading cause of death, and peaked in the 1960s. Since that time the percentage of deaths from heart disease has steadily declined, even after adjusting for changes in the ways that diseases have been classified and diagnosed, and adjusting for the growing proportion of elderly in the population. The decline has touched males and females, whites and nonwhites.

Estimated Actual Benefit of Interventions on Coronary Heart Disease Mortality Rates, 1968–76

	Estimated lives saved	Estimated decline in mortality
Medical interventions		
Coronary care units	85,000	13.5%
Prehospital resuscitation and care	25,000	4.0%
Coronary artery bypass surgery	23,000	3.5%
Medical treatment of clinical coronary heart disease	61,000	10.0%
Treatment of hypertension	55,000	8.5%
Total	249,000	39.5%
Changes in life style		
Reduction in serum cholesterol levels	190,000	30.0%
Reduction in cigarette smoking	150,000	24.0%
Total	340,000	54.0%
Not explained or due to errors in preceding estimates	41,000	6.5%
Total lives saved	630,000	—

In 1985 the absolute number of deaths caused by heart disease in the United States was 541,000, similar to the number in 1963; however, because the nation's population was larger, the incidence was actually lower. If death rates had remained what they were in 1963, we would have expected 898,000 deaths from coronary heart disease in 1985—a difference of 357,000 deaths in that year alone.

In fact, we owe to epidemiologic methods our confidence that the decline in heart disease is real, and not just a consequence of changes in reporting, and our understanding of which changes or programs contributed to the decline. In 1978, and again in 1986, the National Heart, Lung and Blood Institute met to assess the decline in coronary heart disease and to consider explanations. Improved management of hypertension and changes in life style, particularly reductions in serum cholesterol levels and cigarette smoking, may explain more than 54 percent of the decline in mortality. Medical care of patients through the use of coronary care units, prehospital resuscitation and care, coronary artery bypass surgery, and medical treatment of coronary heart disease explained another 31 percent of the decline.

Only rough estimates can be made of the quantitative contribution of each new tactic to the overall decline in mortality from heart disease. It is difficult to compare the effect of food labeling to the effect of hypertension management or to the effect of coronary artery bypass surgery. Even more difficult is the evaluation of their cost-effectiveness. While diagnostic and treatment procedures have come into increased use in the last several decades, they have also consumed more health care dollars, an issue we discuss in greater detail in Chapter 8.

The dramatic and persistent decline in mortality from heart disease of the last thirty years may represent epidemiology's successful encounter with an epidemic of chronic disease. Epidemiologic studies have identified risk factors for heart disease, developed programs for preventing the disease, and evaluated treatments for heart disease and the related conditions of hypertension and hypercholesterolemia. In so doing, they have contributed to the development of important tools—the concept of risk factor, multivariable analysis, randomized clinical trials, and cohort studies—that have enriched the field of epidemiology itself.

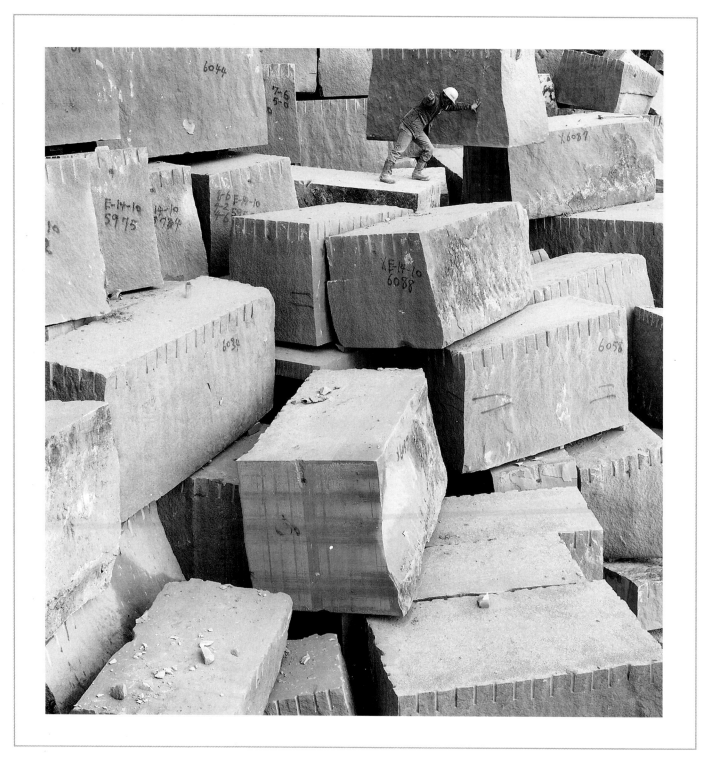

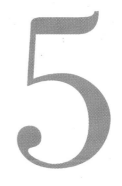

Hazards in the Environment: Finding "Safe" Levels

STONES FOR buildings and monuments must be quarried, cut, and finished. Each process produces dust that endangers the health of the workers involved. One of the tasks of epidemiology has been to determine acceptable levels of exposure to dust and other hazards of the workplace and environment.

The workplace, and indeed the environment in general, has probably been a source of disease for thousands of years. Charles Doughty, an Englishman who traveled in Arabia in the 1870s, described the harm done by the ancient craft of stone cutting in his book *Travels to Arabia Deserta*, first published in 1888:

> Their toil is so noxious (under this breathless climate), that he who in the vigorous hope of his youth is allured by the higher wage to cast in his lot with the stone-hewers may hardly come to ripe years, or even to his middle age. When the sharp flying powder has settled in the lungs, cutting and consuming them as glass, there is no power in Nature which can expel it again—A young stone-hewer came to me; his beard was only beginning to spring, but he was sick unto death: he could not go the length of a few houses. Sheykh Nasir said, "Thus they all perish early; in two or three years they die."

Hazards of the workplace and environment have been the object of scientific scrutiny since the late seventeenth century, when Bernardino Ramazzini first began to systematically study diseases as they are related to occupation. Several developments in our own century have led to more intense studies of environmental and occupational exposures. Industrialization has increased the number of hazardous materials that are produced, used, and ultimately discarded in our environment, while population growth has multiplied the quantities of materials produced and the numbers of people affected. At the same time, today's environmental hazards are not accepted as passively as those faced by the Arabian stone-cutters: labor movements have agitated for protection of workers' health; and the public has demanded a cleaner, safer environment. Epidemiology has been a major tool used to describe hazards, document their effects on health, and set rational guidelines for safety in both the workplace and the environment.

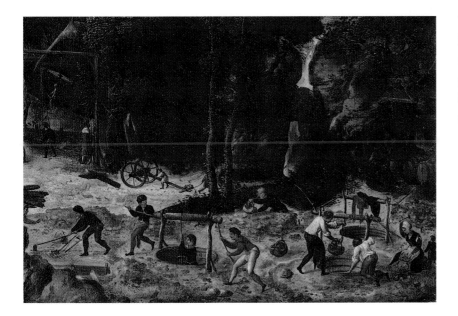

The ancient activity of mining has always been a hazardous occupation. The copper miners depicted in this sixteenth-century painting by Herri met de Bles could have been exposed to silica dust from chipped rock.

Like other epidemiologic research, occupational and environmental epidemiology aims to assess an exposure to a hazardous substance and determine if it causes the disease in question. But, unlike other areas of epidemiologic research, we are often certain that the exposure causes disease and are instead concerned with quantifying dangerous levels of exposure. Harmful exposures often cannot be totally eliminated from the workplace or the environment, and much occupational and environmental research is aimed at determining a safe or acceptable level of a dangerous exposure. The inherent contradiction in finding a "safe" level for a dangerous exposure generates much debate, and it becomes essential to obtain precise measures of the amount of exposure, or "dose." Can there be acceptable exposures to air pollution, radiation, asbestos, and so on? What levels are permissible, and what doses unacceptable?

Questions that are difficult to answer scientifically become even more difficult to resolve politically when safety must be balanced against economic cost to the public in tax expenditures, loss of jobs, or loss of products. Occupational and environmental epidemiology quickly gives rise to issues of public policy that are of concern to most citizens and thus relevant well beyond the scientific community.

Of many possible examples we have chosen two to explore in detail. The following stories of asbestos and lead as focuses of epidemiological investigation reveal both the crucial scope of such research and key stages in the evolution of the discipline.

Asbestos: Occupational Epidemiology Describes a Widespread Health Hazard

ASBESTOS is one of several minerals now known to cause lung diseases in people who inhale the dust. The diseases are named after the minerals or agents that cause the disease: asbestosis, byssinosis, silicosis, siderosis (in iron workers), anthracosis (in coal workers), and so forth. These dusts cause disease by acting as physical irritants in the lungs and injuring lung tissue, but some dusts also increase the lung's susceptibility to cancer and other lung diseases and some, like asbestos, are themselves carcinogens, causing cancer in people who inhale or swallow the material.

The history of asbestosis follows the history of asbestos—its mining, processing, and use in hundreds of applications. In the years from 1857 to 1880, asbestos began being used in sealings and packings; in 1866 a material was developed from it for heat insulation, and many diverse products followed. Physicians began reporting cases of pulmonary fibrosis (a fibrous thickening of the lungs) in asbestos workers at the turn of the century. The oldest documented case is that reported by H. Montagu-Murray in 1906 based on an autopsy performed in 1899. Other deaths among asbestos workers were reported but attributed to lime dust, lead exposure, or tuberculosis; occupational lung diseases were often confused with tuberculosis (silicosis; another example of such a disease is discussed in the box on pages 114–115). In 1924 and 1927 W. E. Cooke and his colleagues described extensive fibrosis in the lungs of a 33-year-old woman who had worked twenty years in asbestos factories. They coined the word "asbestosis," but it was several years before the disease was fully recognized.

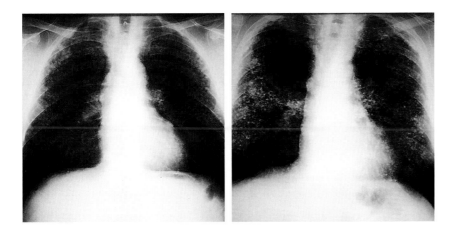

X-rays reveal two stages in the course of silicosis. From left to right: stage 1, the lungs of a furnace cleaner and sand blaster exposed for 23 years to silica dust; stage 2, the lungs of a mason exposed for 24 years.

Researchers in 1935 began observing cases of lung cancer among asbestos workers with and without asbestosis; they observed the first case of mesothelioma, a rare malignant tumor of the surface lining of the lung, in an asbestos worker in 1947. The task of epidemiologists was to sort out the role of asbestos in each of these diseases, describe the interrelationships between the diseases (does asbestosis increase one's susceptibility to lung cancer and to mesothelioma?), and recommend acceptable levels of exposure.

To describe the relationship between asbestos exposure and each of the diseases—asbestosis, lung cancer, and mesothelioma—epidemiologists needed to adapt the infectious model of causality to the study of occupational and environmental disease, as had been done for cancer and heart disease. One postulate in establishing the pathogenic cause of disease is that the organism causing the disease should be able to be cultured from a person having the disease. An analogous requirement for a dust exposure would be that the dust be found in the patient's tissues. But dust is often metabolized or excreted even while in the act of

Silicosis

Silicosis, like asbestosis, is a lung disease named for the mineral dust that causes it. Miners and stonecutters are especially at risk because they are constantly exposed to silica dust during quarrying, cutting or finishing stone. Dust inhalation has long been recognized as a hazard, but in the wake of the discovery that tuberculosis is caused by a bacterium, the medical establishment was nonetheless slow to recognize silicosis as a separate medical entity. The presence of lung disease among poor miners or stonecutters was consistent with the distribution of tuberculosis; indeed, many workers with silicosis also had tuberculosis. Therefore it was relatively easy to disregard the occupational cause of phthisis (another turn-of-the-century term for "consumption," the wasting away associated with lung disease) and to maintain that silicosis was a form of tuberculosis.

The medical and public health communities may have been slow to recognize occupational causes of disease, but the insurance industry readily understood the health risks associated with mining. Frederick L. Hoffman, a statistician and later vice president at the Prudential Life Insurance Company, conducted painstaking studies in town after town, collecting information from physicians, coroners, local libraries, graveyards, and employers. He visited the worksites in each

town to document the health risks of employees. He then developed actuarial charts and made recommendations to Prudential about which groups of workers to insure. Despite the very pragmatic application of his work, Hoffman also generalized from his findings and synthesized a coherent argument supporting the theory that dust could cause lung disease even in the absence of bacteria. He published his work in the medical, occupational, and government literature, providing a basis for future work in occupational health.

Hoffman did not consider himself an epidemiologist; from 1908 to 1922, the main years in which he published, epidemiologists were busy tracking down contagious diseases. Nonetheless, from our present-day perspective, we can readily appreciate his classic epidemiologic approach: the careful accrual of information; the tabulation and counting of events; comparisons between groups; and the building of a body of evidence that forms a logical argument in favor of a biological theory of disease causation. Hoffman was able to use this approach to support his conclusion that

the destructive effects of the dust-laden atmosphere of factories and workshops are a decided serious menace to health and life. . . . Dust in any form, when inhaled continuously

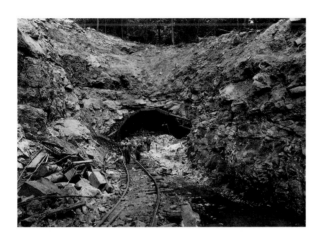

The Hawk's Nest Tunnel, West Virginia, was built in the early 1930s by digging through solid silica rock. The intense exposure to silica dust may have resulted in over 700 deaths among the men who dug the tunnel.

and in considerable quantities, is prejudicial to health because of its inherent mechanical properties, destructive to the delicate membrane of the respiratory passages and the lungs.

Workers knew that dust from digging tunnels was killing them. In 1936 the renowned blues singer Josh White, using the pseudonym Pinewood Tom, wrote and recorded a song about the Hawk's Nest Tunnel called "Silicosis Is Killing Me."

I said, "Silicosis, you made a mighty bad break of me,
Oh, Silicosis, you made a mighty bad break of me,
You robbed me of my youth and health,
All you brought poor me was misery.
Now, Silicosis, you dirty robber and a thief,
Robbed me of my right to live,
And all you brought to me was grief."
I was there diggin' that tunnel for six bits a day,
Didn't know I was diggin' my own grave.
Silicosis eatin' my lungs away.
I says, "Mama, Mama, Mama, cool my fevered head,"
I says, "Mama, Mama, cool my fevered head,
I'm gonna leave my Jesus, God knows I'll soon be dead."
Six bits I got for diggin', diggin' that tunnel hole.
Take me away from my baby,
It sho' done wrecked my soul.
Now tell all my buddies, tell all my friends you see.
I'm going way up yonder.
Please don't weep for me. ●

causing disease and long before the expression of clinical symptoms. Instead of using the Koch-Henle postulates, Irving Selikoff, a pioneer investigator of the health hazards of asbestos, adapted the Bradford Hill criteria of causality (the same criteria used in assessing the relationship between smoking and lung cancer) to occupational epidemiology, stipulating:

1. That a statistically significant association be established between exposures of persons to the agent and the subsequent development of the syndrome (strength of association).
2. That correspondence be established between the extent of exposure and the extent of the appearance of essential elements of the syndrome; i.e., that at least some degree of dose-response relationship be demonstrable.
3. That, in the event that the agent or its metabolic product can be demonstrated in tissue, its concentration in diseased persons should be greater than that in non-diseased persons.
4. That the demonstration of pathological changes in an animal following exposure to the agent, similar to those seen in human beings, would strengthen the evidence for causation, but that failure to obtain such changes would not necessarily negate other evidence supporting a causative relationship (biological plausibility).
5. That the role of numerous attendant circumstances capable of influencing the appearance or manifestations of the disease initiated by the agent in question should be evaluated.

Selikoff wrote further: "Under these circumstances, proof of a causal relationship depends on the weight of the evidence rather than a demonstration of complete conformity to all five postulates." Thus the evidence for the association between asbestos and asbestosis, lung cancer, and mesothelioma had to be accumulated in a painstaking way to satisfy each of the five criteria and to determine the levels of exposure associated with disease. Occupational disease may develop over time and repeated exposure; several diseases may develop, and some diseases may develop many years after exposure. The evidence regarding occupational exposure and

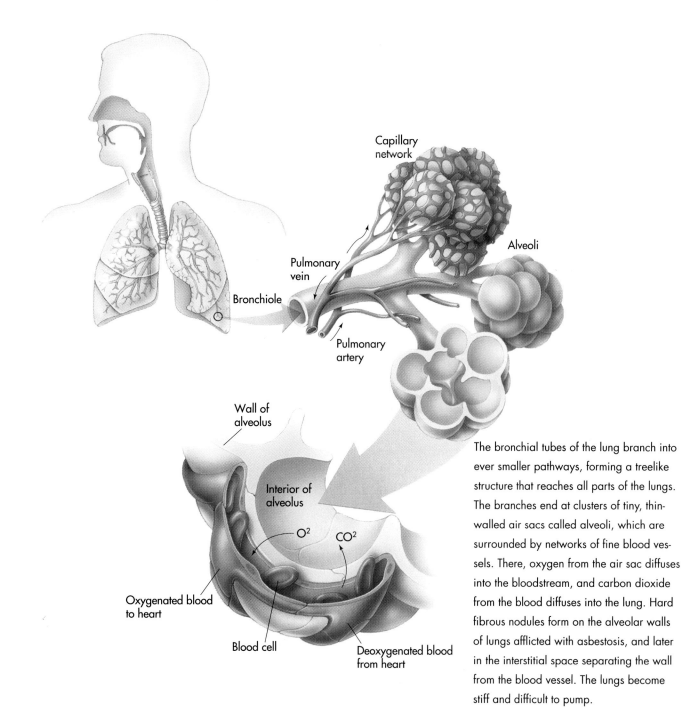

Capillary
network

Alveoli

Pulmonary
vein

Bronchiole

Pulmonary
artery

Wall of
alveolus

Interior of
alveolus

O^2 CO^2

Oxygenated blood
to heart

Blood cell

Deoxygenated blood
from heart

The bronchial tubes of the lung branch into
ever smaller pathways, forming a treelike
structure that reaches all parts of the lungs.
The branches end at clusters of tiny, thin-
walled air sacs called alveoli, which are
surrounded by networks of fine blood vessels. There, oxygen from the air sac diffuses
into the bloodstream, and carbon dioxide
from the blood diffuses into the lung. Hard
fibrous nodules form on the alveolar walls
of lungs afflicted with asbestosis, and later
in the interstitial space separating the wall
from the blood vessel. The lungs become
stiff and difficult to pump.

disease may be complex, and the "weighing" of such complex evidence may seem less than tidy.

Asbestosis was defined as a lung condition caused by exposure to asbestos; the question of causality did not arise in the same way as for smoking and lung cancer. Instead, the crucial questions were: How much asbestos exposure could cause asbestosis (and how could a worker document his or her level of exposure in legal claims)? How much exposure to asbestos in the workplace or community is acceptable? These questions translated into questions regarding the causal relationship between a specified level of exposure and disease: i.e., Do x years of exposure to y levels of asbestos *cause* asbestosis (or lung cancer, or mesothelioma)?

Defining the Danger: Estimating Levels of Exposure

THE association between asbestos exposure and asbestosis was clear in the 1930s. Various studies estimated that from 12 to 53 percent of asbestos workers in that decade showed pulmonary fibrosis or moderate asbestosis. Investigators could demonstrate a dose-response relationship by establishing that the longer people worked with or around asbestos, the more likely they were to develop the lung disease. The "dose" could be defined according to (1) the number of years of exposure, (2) the intensity of exposure, or (3) a combined measure of both length of employment and intensity of exposure. Looking at workers by the number of years employed where there was an asbestos exposure, one could see the severity of the disease, as well as the proportion of workers afflicted with the disease increasing. The number of years of exposure was a measure of the amount of exposure, but it was also a reflection of the time needed for disease to develop.

Crude efforts to categorize exposure into heavy or light, continuous or intermittent, or work environments as less dusty or more dusty, showed that more intense exposure led to higher incidence of disease. Such comparative categories, however, did not provide information about actual levels.

The measurement of dust and other occupational and environmental exposures has emerged as a subspecialty of this area of epidemiology. Measuring asbestos particles in the air presents technical challenges be-

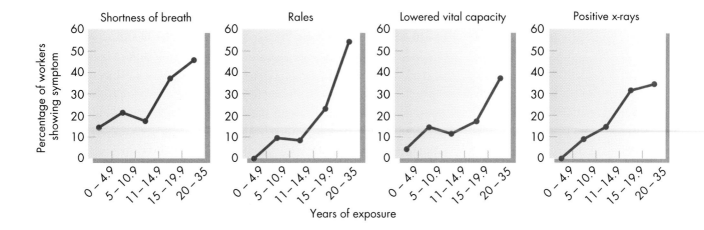

Years of exposure

cause of variations in fiber size, fiber shape, or type and composition. The measurement of all occupational exposures is complicated by variations in exposure among individuals, within a workplace, or over job categories, and by use of safety equipment or engineering controls. Moreover, exposure may vary over time as methods and workplace procedures change. Workers sometimes wear devices that measure exposure immediately nearby and provide quantified personal measurements. A photosensitive film badge to measure exposure to radioactivity is one example of an unobtrusive device designed to not affect an individual's behavior (but which may be left on the lab coat on the back of a chair, rather than with the worker). Other monitoring devices may be more cumbersome and limit a worker's normal range of activities. Measurements of exposure within a defined area may be easier to collect, but may not reflect the actual exposure experienced by individuals. Another option is to rank job titles by their estimated overall levels of exposure.

Safety practices, such as ventilation or hosing down of dust, can reduce an individual's exposure, as can the wearing of respirators or other protective equipment. It is more difficult to measure the dose that the worker actually receives than to measure the concentration of an exposure in the worker's immediate environment. Biological monitoring of blood, urine, or breath may allow estimates of the burden experienced by individual workers.

A study of 101 pipe coverers exposed to asbestos found that the percentage of workers showing the symptoms of lung disease increased as their number of years of exposure rose.

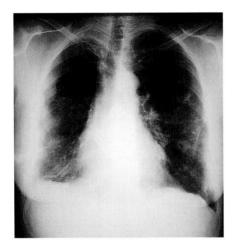

The lungs of a worker exposed to raw asbestos fiber for ten years, when x-rayed, show areas of calcified tissue.

When studying the effect of occupational exposures on disease, an investigator can track how the exposure affects the health of workers as time passes, or study the exposure history of workers whose health is currently known. The advantage of the first approach, a prospective cohort study, is that one may take accurate and objective exposure measurements; the disadvantage is that the disease may take ten, twenty, or more years to develop. The investigator may have to wait a long time to see the relationship between exposure and disease.

The alternative approach is to estimate exposure levels from historical records and to compare workers' exposure histories to their present-day health status. Two study designs can be used: the case-control study and the reconstructed cohort study. Both these designs allow an investigator to evaluate the relationship between exposure and disease without waiting twenty or thirty years for results. In a case-control study of occupational disease, one identifies cases of the disease of interest, then compares the exposure histories of those affected to the histories of workers without the disease. In a reconstructed cohort study, one identifies the entire group of workers who began work in a plant, industry, job category, or occupation during a specified time period. One then describes their exposure histories and compares the health of workers, including the presence of various diseases, in each exposure category. The reconstructed cohort study allows the investigator to compare the experiences of workers with different durations of employment, as well as to compare the occurrence of more than one disease. Essential to both designs are methods of assessing historical exposures and making inferences that are relevant to the present-day work environment.

Investigators rely on a variety of sources to reconstruct exposure histories. In some industries, efforts to measure exposure have been in place for several decades. Plant records of inspections or required monitoring can provide data such as particles per unit of air, but such overall measurements may not describe an individual's level of exposure. Although personal monitors (for example, badges recording exposure to radiation) have been used for several decades in industries where exposure to radiation is suspected, most other occupational work sites have not monitored personal exposure levels. Sometimes, records of plant production, sched-

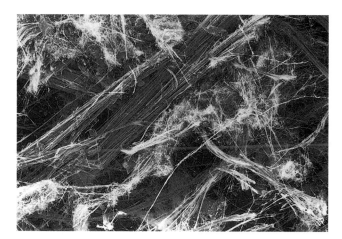

A false-color scanning electron micrograph of fibers of crocidolite, one of the common varieties of asbestos. Like all asbestos varieties, crocidolite is a silicate. Asbestos fibers can be compressed, felted, or woven to make insulating boards, paper, and shingles.

ules, and shipments may indicate when new materials were handled and produced and can suggest times of high exposure. The problem faced by investigators is to estimate an individual's exposure from general data collected at a plant. One solution is to compare detailed work histories with information about the exposures in specific job categories and work areas.

The work of John Dement and his colleagues at the University of North Carolina at Chapel Hill illustrates how painstaking a process estimating individual exposure levels can be. In 1983 the team published their study assessing exposure levels among workers at a plant that began producing asbestos packing materials for steam engines and pumps in 1896, and asbestos textiles in 1909. Although only one type of raw fiber asbestos (called chrysotile) had been used in the plant, the team's assessment was complicated by the fact that small amounts of an asbestos yarn (called crocidolite) had also been used from the 1950s to 1975 to make braided packings. The researchers had to consider all sources of asbestos in their estimates of exposure. Their work illustrates the necessity of understanding the history of a particular plant and industry; since factory activities change over time, exposures may not be constant.

Studies conducted by the U.S. Public Health Service in January and February of 1937 had described the plant practices as "representative of the best practice in the country at this time." The plant owners had added local exhaust ventilation and requested an industrial hygiene study in

Summary of Exposure Estimates for Fiber Preparation and Waste Recovery Operation

Uniform job category	Estimated mean fiber exposures (fibers > 5 μm/cc)		
	1930–44	1945–64	1965–75
General area personnel	26.2	8.1	5.8
Machine operators			
Fly machine operator	78.0	23.9	17.2
Crusher operator	78.0	23.9	—
Waste machine operator	45.9	14.1	10.1
Clean-up personnel	54.4	16.7	12.0
Raw fiber handling	35.0	10.8	7.3

November 1937. These documents enabled researchers in the 1980s to estimate the overall levels of dust in the plant at that time. Detective work involving Public Health Service documents and insurance, state, and plant engineering records helped researchers reconstruct a history of engineering controls in the factory during the years from 1930 to 1975 and changes in overall dust levels.

To document each individual worker's exposure, the researchers began by collecting data about each job at the factory, the years the job was in existence, and the exposure levels for each job. The factory was categorized into zones representing different levels of exposure. Within each zone, workers were assigned job categories as follows: (1) general area personnel (service personnel, fixers, oilers), (2) machine operation, (3) cleanup, and (4) raw fiber handling. The team developed mathematical formulas to take into account for each job title, the type of work, average exposure, and time spent in a particular zone. The results were tables such as the one on this page, which estimate exposure levels for job categories and their changes over time. The final step was to reconstruct individual worker histories; by looking at the calendar years each job was held, the length of time at each job, and the exposure levels for each job, the team could estimate individual exposures to asbestos.

Such calculations were carried out for 1,261 white males employed for one or more months in textile production, with at least one month falling between 1940 and 1965. The researchers examined death certificates in 1975 for the causes of any deaths in the group. Thus, each worker began exposure before 1965 and had until 1975 to die from the disease—a minimum of ten years between exposure and outcome, as is required by studies of diseases with long latency periods.

The researchers observed 308 deaths, but 206 of these would have been expected in any similarly aged group of white men living between 1940 and 1965 (based on national mortality statistics). Comparing observed deaths to expected deaths produced a measure, the standardized mortality ratio, of (308/206) $\times$ 100 or 150—indicating that the number of deaths was 50 percent higher than expected. The dose-relationship was strong: those at the lowest level of exposure showed an approximately 40 percent increase in risk of lung cancer, whereas those at the highest levels showed a risk 18 times greater than expected.

The level of detail attained by Dement and his colleagues greatly strengthened their evidence linking asbestos exposure and lung disease. A less thorough measurement of exposure would have left more room to question their findings. Their painstaking accrual of data bears a striking similarity to Snow's efforts in his investigation of the cholera epidemic of 1854. In Dement's study, however, the methods of epidemiology were used to accumulate evidence regarding the "epidemic" of asbestos-related disease.

Asbestos concentrations were first expressed in million particles per cubic foot, and later as fibers per cubic centimeter, as is the current practice. As early as 1938, studies in asbestos textile mills led researchers to recommend a standard of no more than 5 million particles of dust per cubic foot of air to prevent asbestosis. This recommendation became law in 1960, 22 years later. In 1969, the federal standard became 12 fibers longer than 5 microns (millionths of a meter) per cubic centimeter of air (thought to be equivalent to 2 million particles per cubic foot of air). The 1969 standard counted only fibers longer than 5 microns in length because few labs were equipped to count smaller fibers. In 1971 the standard was tightened to allow only 5 fibers per cubic centimeter, with the

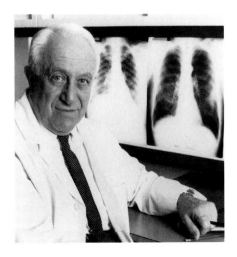

Irving Selikoff, whose work was instrumental in documenting the hazards of asbestos.

goal of reduction to 2 fibers in 1976. A standard of 0.2 was implemented in the late 1980s. This trend toward more stringent standards is the result of epidemiologic studies that can discriminate between finer and finer levels of exposure, and can also be seen in other areas of occupational and environmental health.

New Dangers from Asbestos

THE first standards regarding asbestos were aimed at preventing asbestosis, but as a reduction in asbestos levels resulted in a lower incidence of that disease, researchers were able to discern such equally serious dangers as lung cancer and mesothelioma, not previously apparent on account of the overwhelming presence of asbestosis and because of the long latency period preceding the development of cancer.

The first case of lung cancer associated with asbestos was reported in 1935. As early as 1941, investigators had found three reasons to believe that asbestos exposure caused lung cancer: (1) 12 to 20 percent of autopsies of asbestos workers showed pulmonary carcinoma; (2) asbestos workers with lung cancer were younger than other lung cancer patients; and (3) their lesions appeared in a different part of the lungs (the lower lobes, rather than the upper lobes affected in people not exposed to asbestos).

The presence of asbestosis in a worker often masked the onset of carcinoma, but studies throughout the 1950s increasingly showed an association between asbestos exposure and lung cancer. During the 1960s and 1970s, Irving Selikoff and his colleagues collected data on four cohorts of asbestos workers. They compared the observed rates of pulmonary carcinoma to the rates that would be expected based on the rates for each age group in the general population. The four cohorts experienced 5.3 times the incidence of lung cancer expected; the ratio of observed rates to expected rates ranged from 3.2 to 7.6. Selikoff's first adapted criterion of causality (that there be an association between exposure and disease) was satisfied.

Lung cancer did not seem to increase with intensity of asbestos exposure, but rather with *duration* of exposure and hence with the cumulative exposure to asbestos dust. Thus the second criterion, that there be a dose-response relationship, may have been satisfied. The third criterion, that the agent be found in the affected tissue, had not been sufficiently studied in people with lung cancer and asbestos exposure but without asbestosis. Animal studies had shown that inhalation of asbestos fibers can cause lung tumors in rats; this satisfied Selikoff's fourth criterion of causality, the development of an animal model.

Selikoff's fifth criterion is that the role of other causal factors be examined, and in the relationship between asbestos and lung cancer the other important causal factor is cigarette smoking. Smoking increases a person's risk of lung cancer about elevenfold, and exposure to asbestos increases the risk of lung cancer about fivefold. In the combined presence of smoking and asbestos exposure, researchers have observed a 55 times increased risk of lung cancer. The separate effects of asbestos and cigarette smoking appear to multiply each other (a multiplicative model) rather than simply add to each other (in an additive model one would expect to see an effect of about 16).

The findings of occupational epidemiologists ultimately suggested that very low levels of asbestos exposure increased a person's risk of asbestosis, lung cancer, and mesothelioma. While asbestos had formerly been thought of as a hazard only in industries manufacturing or using asbestos products, evidence showing a relationship between lower levels of asbestos exposure and disease suggested that building materials like wallboard, insulation, and cement products may expose the entire population to the hazards of asbestos in their homes, schools, and offices. The result was the creation of governmental regulations aimed at removing asbestos hazards from public buildings. The findings from occupational epidemiology, thus, were useful in informing issues of environmental epidemiology.

Lead: The Modern Investigation of an Ancient Hazard

SOME of the dangers of excessive lead exposure have been known for hundreds of years, but modern epidemiology has added to that knowledge by describing in detail the many adverse effects of lower levels of lead ex-

The Cholic, engraved by George Cruikshank in 1819, depicts the violent inward contractions of lead cholic as the pulling of a rope surrounding the victim's body. The symptoms of severe lead poisoning were well known for centuries. Such severe lead poisoning no longer occurs, and modern epidemiology has described the symptoms of lower and lower levels of lead exposure.

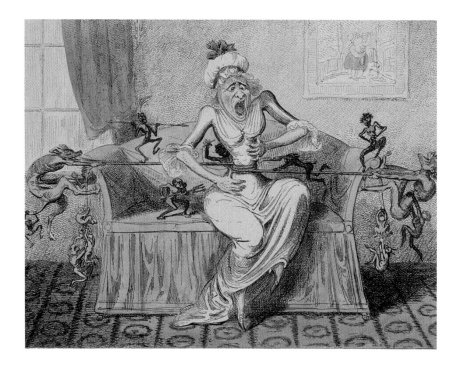

posure, and, by identifying the routes of exposure, it has spurred regulation of the lead content of paint, gasoline, and cook- and dinnerware.

The first law in North America regulating lead exposure may have been the law passed by the Massachusetts Bay Colony in 1723 that forbade the use of lead pipes or materials containing lead in the distillation of rum. Some sixty years later Benjamin Franklin recalled the passage of this law as his first awareness of the dangers of lead exposure. He had also been warned not to warm his printing types because of the lead fumes given off, and he would not drink rainwater that had dripped off a roof painted with lead-based paint. Dry bellyache, *colica pictonum,* and dry gripes were some of the names used to describe the stomach pains and constipation associated with the ingestion of large quantities of lead. In 1767 a Dr. Baker solved the mystery of "Devonshire colic." He discovered that exclusively in the English region of Devonshire, millstones in apple presses were hewn in segments and bound together with molten lead. The lead leached into the cider, a favorite beverage in Devonshire, and caused the local colic.

In 1786, Benjamin Franklin wrote a letter to his friend Benjamin Vaughn (Secretary to Lord Shelburne in England) about the dangers of lead. He concluded with the statement, "You will observe with concern how long a useful truth may be known and exist, before it is generally receiv'd and practic'd on." If the dangers of lead ingestion were well known in the eighteenth century, what did modern epidemiology add to this knowledge? The colic noticed in the 1700s was a result of high levels of lead exposure, greater than 50 mg/dl in the blood. In the twentieth century, epidemiologists documented the adverse effects of ever lower levels of lead exposure, and their work led to a reexamination of all our guidelines concerning lead exposure.

The acute neurological symptoms of lead poisoning, such as coma or convulsions, were also well known by the 1800s, but 1930s texts on lead poisoning erroneously stated that its neurological effects were reversible and generally subsided after removal from exposure. The work of Randolph Byers and Elizabeth Lord in 1943 first showed that even years after the symptoms of acute lead poisoning had subsided, children's performance in school was severely impaired. Byers and Lord gathered records on 20 children treated for lead poisoning at ages one to five and looked at their school performances at ages six to twelve. The researchers considered 18 and possibly 19 of the children to have failed in school; that is, the children had been expelled, showed severe sensorimotor deficits, or had repeated grades.

From 1930 through the 1960s health workers focused their efforts on identifying cases of lead poisoning. It appeared to occur mostly in old cities among children of ages one to six residing in dilapidated housing; the children ate chips of lead-based paint or ingested lead in dust in the course of their normal activities. A late-awakened consciousness of the problem led to mass screening programs in the 1970s. While 25 to 45 percent of children in "high risk" areas of Chicago and New York showed evidence of undue lead absorption, lead exposure was also found in unexpected populations, among urban and rural children of all income levels.

Wrist drop is an extreme clinical symptom of nerve damage caused by lead exposure; mottled teeth can also result from excessive exposure to lead. Such high levels of exposure are rarely seen anymore, although lead is still a hazard.

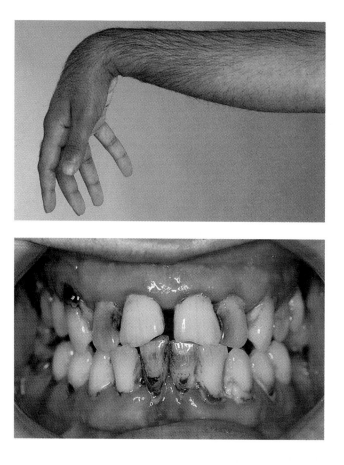

Epidemiologists then directed their efforts in two directions: (1) toward identifying the sources of lead exposure and (2) toward correlating exposure levels with health effects. Ingestion of lead-based paint remained the most important source of high lead exposure, but leaded gasoline, lead-soldered cans, lead dust brought home by parents exposed to lead at work, proximity to lead smelting plants and battery reclamation plants—all resulted in lead exposure.

While investigators were identifying multiple sources of lead exposure, they were also discovering that lead exposure had negative health effects at exposure levels far lower than those that caused acute episodes of lead poisoning. In the 1970s Herbert Needleman and his colleagues, examining children with lower levels of lead exposure than those previously studied, found psychological and behavioral problems. They used a technique that allowed them to measure long-term exposure: instead of measuring blood levels, they measured the lead found in children's baby teeth as the teeth were naturally shed. The teeth of 2,335 children were measured for lead, and the children were classified into six levels of lead exposure. Teachers, who were kept ignorant of their students' lead levels, were asked to rate the children on eleven characteristics: distractibility, ability to stick to a task, organization, hyperactivity, "daydreaming," and the like. When the teachers' ratings were plotted against the lead levels, a clear, consistent dose-response was found. As lead exposure increased, neuropsychological problems increased, even though all the lead levels were below those previously thought to be harmful.

By asking teachers to rate their students on eleven classroom behaviors and by measuring lead levels in teeth, Herbert Needleman was able to document that small increases in lead exposure were correlated with a variety of emotional and behavioral problems in school children.

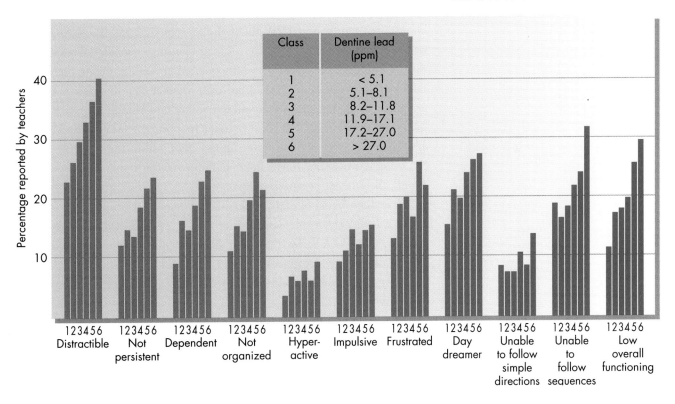

Class	Dentine lead (ppm)
1	< 5.1
2	5.1–8.1
3	8.2–11.8
4	11.9–17.1
5	17.2–27.0
6	> 27.0

More recent studies have detected unfortunate neuropsychological effects at lead levels as low as 10 to 15 μg/dl (the unit μg, short for microgram, represents one millionth of a gram). Such low levels of exposure may be common in the population—the second National Health and Nutrition Examination Survey in 1976–80 found average blood lead levels of 10 to 18 μg/dl, with a range from 2.0 to almost 70.0. Measurements of the lead in umbilical cord blood have demonstrated that even in the uterus the fetus may be exposed to lead. Such exposures have been found to be predictive of minor malformations and of psychometric intelligence at age two years, after other variables are taken into account. For example, the study of umbilical cord blood levels and malformations also measured smoking, alcohol use, drugs, and past health history and used statistical techniques to measure the contribution of all these other variables.

These and other studies gave epidemiologists more detailed knowledge about the adverse effects of different levels of lead exposure. New knowledge, too, was gained about the effects of lead exposures in the workplace. As a result, the level of lead exposure considered acceptable was lowered in both industry and the home. For lead in the air, the official permissible exposure of 200 μg/m^3 over eight hours on average was established by OSHA (the Occupational Safety and Health Administration) in 1971. In 1973, NIOSH (the National Institute for Occupational Safety and Health) recommended lowering the permissible limit to 150 μg/m^3. By 1978, OSHA had recommended reducing the limit over time to 50 μg/m^3, the current permissible level.

Scientists had originally thought that lead poisoning occurred only above a threshold level. Research of the 1970s and 1980s led to a new paradigm. We now know that lead exposure occurs along a continuum, and so do the adverse effects of lead exposure; there is no level of lead exposure that can be considered a threshold or dividing line below which exposure is safe.

One of the reasons for this shift is that researchers began looking at outcomes that could be measured on continuous scales (such as I.Q.) instead of health effects (such as lead poisoning) that were categorized dichotomously. When Needleman and others began to look at neuropsycho-

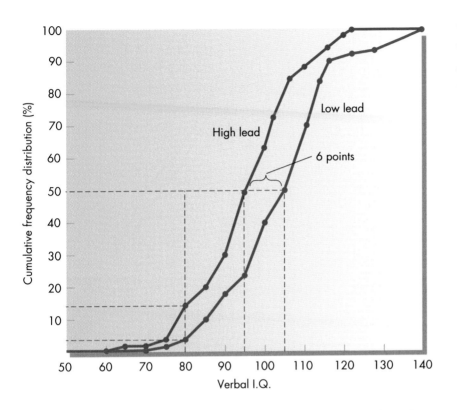

How important is a six-point difference in I.Q.? A six-point shift in the average I.Q. can produce a fourfold increase in the number of people whose I.Q. is under 80 (considered to be a severe deficit).

logical traits that were distributed along a continuum, they could pick up the effects of lower levels of exposure and demonstrate that the effects occurred at *every* level of lead exposure. Finding differences in neuropsychological traits, society then had to decide whether these effects were acceptable.

How important was a six-point difference in the median I.Q. of exposed and less exposed subjects? Such a shift in the I.Q. curve would result in a fourfold increase in the number of people with I.Q.s below 80, considered a severe deficit. Epidemiologists can describe such a change, but the public must decide if it is an acceptable consequence of previously set lead-exposure levels.

Efforts to reduce lead exposure were complicated by the many sources of lead. While lead paint remained the main source of acute lead poisoning in children, gasoline with lead additives released lead into the atmosphere, so that the entire population was exposed to lead in the air

Removing lead from gasoline appears to have decreased blood lead levels.

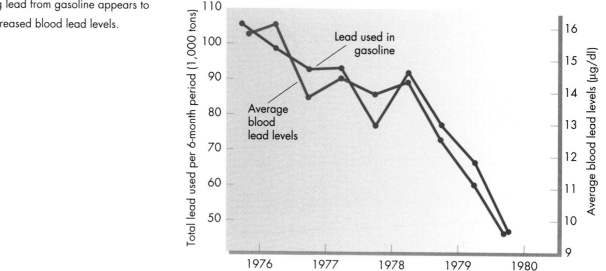

they breathed. The 1970 Clean Air Act provided that the Environmental Protection Agency set safe levels of exposure for all known pollutants. The proposed safe level for lead was 2 $\mu g/m^3$, but agency data showed that millions of people were exposed to airborne lead levels in excess of this level.

Tap water may be a source of lead even when there are no lead pipes, since lead solder in copper pipes and other sources of lead may elevate lead levels in the water. In 1985 the EPA recommended lowering the maximum allowable lead concentration in tap water from 50 to 20 $\mu g/l$, but the mean concentration of lead in tap water remained 29 $\mu g/l$. The EPA estimated that 42 million Americans drank tap water with lead levels above the acceptable limit. If lead solder in copper pipes can elevate lead levels in the water, it follows that food can be a source of lead because of the water used in food preparation. Dust and soil lead can also contribute to exposure, particularly for children who play in the dirt or mouth objects with dust or dirt on them. In neighborhoods with older housing, flakes or droplets from the many coats of lead paint can accumulate in the soil around older buildings and increase a child's exposure to the substance.

As well as documenting the many sources of lead exposure (besides those linked to occupations), epidemiologists continue to describe other adverse effects of lead. Following a classic pattern of epidemiologic discovery, one physician, Richard P. Wedeen, happened to treat a patient whose case intrigued him and led him to similar cases. In 1971 Wedeen saw a patient, a young man, who had been hospitalized six times in the previous two years because of abdominal pain. Each hospitalization re-

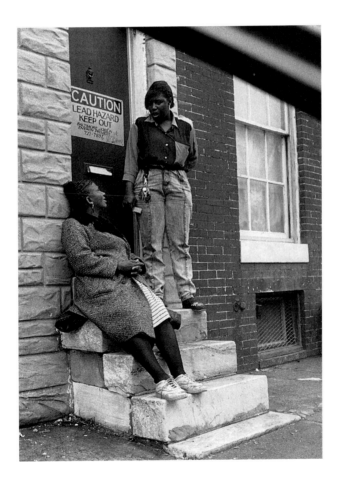

In the 1960s and 1970s, the public became aware of the hazards of lead paint, especially in old, run-down housing, where the lead endangered young children who might chew on or swallow paintchips.

Epidemiology helped to demonstrate that the hazards of lead exposure range along a continuum, instead of being divided by a threshold.

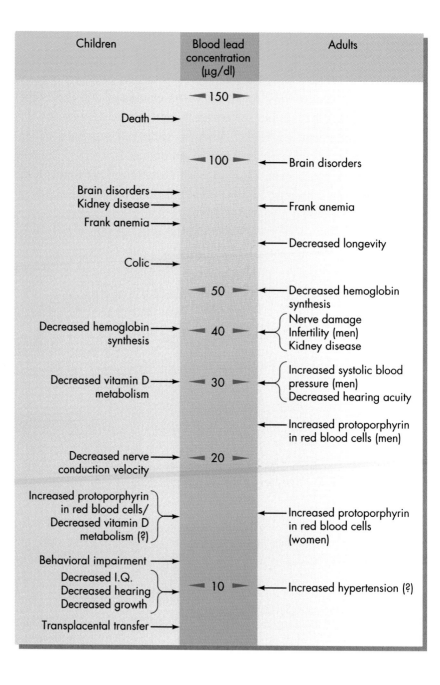

sulted in a different diagnosis: hepatitis, ulcer, gastritis, gall bladder disease, viral infection, and neurosis. Each hospitalization seemed to relieve his pain, but the pains returned one or two months after his return to work. The patient worked preparing solder creams, converting molten lead to powder. One previous physician had suspected lead poisoning, but the patient's blood lead level was below the then-acceptable 80 $\mu g/100$ ml.

Dr. Wedeen chose to measure the effect of lead on the patient's kidney function, using a lead-mobilization test that had been used to study lead nephropathy (kidney damage) in Australia ten years earlier. He not only found evidence of lead poisoning, but also documented a 40 percent decrease in the man's kidney function. Although textbooks and governmental guidelines claimed that kidney diseases due to occupational lead exposure were rare in the United States, Wedeen pursued the detective work so typical of classical epidemiology. He searched for more cases, eventually finding a labor union that allowed him to examine its workers. Out of 30 men examined, 8 had abnormal amounts of lead in their bodies, and 4 of these had unexplained kidney disease. Over five years, Wedeen eventually found 21 cases of unsuspected kidney disease in lead workers. In 15 cases no other cause of disease could be found, and in 4 cases the disease was reversed by long-term chelation therapy: that is, removal of excess body lead stores returned the patients' kidney function to normal.

Other scientists helped document the prevalence of lead nephropathy among lead workers, and occupational standards were revised with the goal of preventing kidney damage in such workers. Another further outcome of this work was that epidemiologists became interested in the potential relationship between lead exposure and hypertension because the toxic effects of lead on the kidney were found to be associated with hypertension and its complications. Analyses of large population databases showed weak but consistent associations between blood lead levels and blood pressure. In 1987 a symposium was held to assess the relationship between lead and blood pressure. At the conclusion of the symposium the argument for causality was assessed as follows:

- The results appear to be *consistent* in different population surveys;
- The *strength of the association* between lead and blood pressure is weak;
- The weak association makes it difficult to assess the presence or absence of a *dose-response relationship;*
- The criterion of *biological plausibility* is partially met (animal evidence supports the hypothesis that lead may cause an increase in blood pressure).

The group used the principles first set forth by Bradford Hill to assess the overall body of evidence regarding the relationship between lead and blood pressure. They concluded by recommending that prospective studies be conducted to study the relationship further.

The consensus among epidemiologists regarding lead and blood pressure was more conservative than the opinions of some lead experts familiar with the many other harmful effects of lead. Epidemiology should be able to act in two ways: to identify a causal relationship where one exists and to point out where causal relationships do not exist or are not yet proven. The question of whether lead is causally related to hypertension is at present undecided.

Asbestos and lead are not the only occupational or environmental exposures that have been studied by epidemiologists, but they are undoubtedly two exposures that have affected millions of people; moreover, resolution of the scientific issues has had a great impact on society. The legal and financial effects are still being felt. Most recently, the New York City school system was unable to open on schedule because asbestos hazards were discovered in school buildings that had been inadequately inspected.

Many scientists may regret that society has been slow in recognizing the dangers of asbestos, lead, and other occupational and environmental exposures. The rate of societal change is an issue that extends beyond the scope of this book, but epidemiology has contributed to the weight of scientific evidence that has made such changes possible by allowing us to base change on solid evidence, to discriminate between strong and weak evidence, and to press for better data where needed.

In environmental and occupational epidemiology, scientific studies are scrutinized by industry, unions, governments, lawyers, and citizens. In the face of these intense pressures, the field of epidemiology has faced unique scientific challenges, particularly the quantitative measurement of exposure and its correlation with effects. Although many materials and occupations have been known to be hazardous for centuries, modern epidemiology has provided more detailed and specific knowledge regarding a range of exposure levels and their varied health effects on the fetus, child, worker, and population at large.

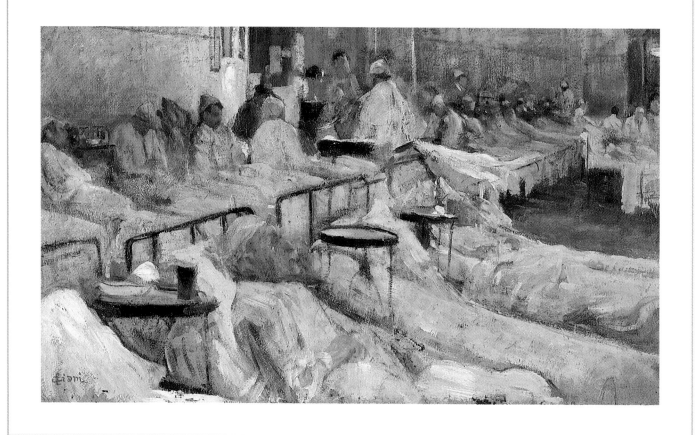

Medicines That Backfire

IN TRYING to do good, a physician may inadvertently do harm. A hospital may be a source of infection, or a drug intended to heal may be a lethal toxin. To determine whether a seemingly reliable therapy is an unsuspected agent of harm, investigators turn to the methods of epidemiology.

Paradoxically, physicians sometimes induce disease in their very efforts to cure it. Diseases and health problems can be caused inadvertently by the same drugs, diagnostic maneuvers, or therapies used by the medical profession to diagnose, treat, and prevent disease. The adjective *iatrogenic* used to describe diseases of this origin comes from ancient Greek roots: *iatros* means "physician" and *genos* means "birth"—hence physician-induced disease. Hippocrates recognized this two-edged sword of medicine when, in the "Oath of Hippocrates," administered to most graduating physicians today, he enjoined his students, "Above all, do no harm." Epidemiology's contribution to the understanding of iatrogenic disease has benefited life and health no less than have its insights into more common types of disease.

In the context of epidemiology, iatrogenic disease comprises the collective unintended negative outcomes of surgical, pharmaceutical, and other interventions—for example, the use of x-ray, ultrasound, CAT, and other imaging technologies—as well as medical therapies. While medical malpractice as a group phenomenon may be a proper focus of epidemiological inquiry, it is important to note that the epidemiologist's concern is with the health of populations. As the stories in this chapter will show, patterns of iatrogenic disease usually reveal not error, but ignorance—of product contamination, rare or delayed side effects, unknown destructive consequences of procedures. Epidemiology observes the pattern, illuminates the possibilities, and seeks the knowledge to remedy or prevent the induced disease.

An early example is that of mid-nineteenth-century physician Ignaz Semmelweis, who noted that the instance of puerperal fever among poor patients in his Vienna hospital population was lower than that of rich women, who received more assiduous medical attention. It became his conviction that physicians were in fact spreading the disease from patient to patient during physical examinations. Simply by insisting that attendants wash their hands well between patients, he sharply diminished the death rate from infection in obstetrical cases. His work anticipated Pasteur's germ theory and Lister's surgical antisepsis—but recognition of his achievement came only decades after contemporary ridicule had driven Semmelweis to madness and suicide.

Many medical detective stories track the iatrogenic spread of infectious disease, and a few have served to reveal flaws in standard surgical procedures—or, more often, to reassess the benefits of certain frequently performed surgeries, from tonsillectomies in the 1950s to hysterectomies and cesarean sections today. The damage caused by misunderstood or mismanufactured drugs provides some particularly compelling examples of medical care gone awry, and epidemiology's efforts on behalf of patients exposed to such drugs is the primary focus of this chapter.

Radiation and Leukemia

WHEN x-ray imaging was first introduced to medical practice at the turn of the century, the dangers of ionizing radiation were not recognized and radiologists were (by present standards) quite careless in their use of this powerful diagnostic and therapeutic tool. Indeed, they commonly placed

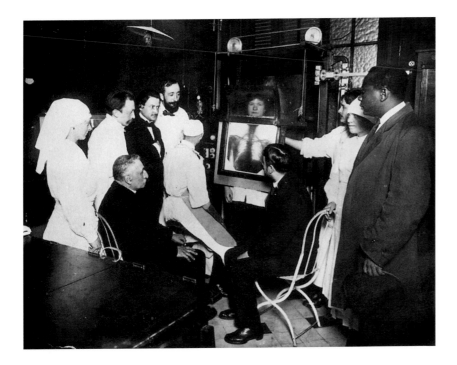

This photograph shows the careless way in which early radiologists handled x-rays: no one is shielded and one of the doctors has his hand in the x-ray field.

their bodies, especially their hands, in the direct path of the radiation. The inevitable appearance of serious skin lesions after some lapse of time eventually led radiologists to take precautions, but it was not until 1975 that a published report conclusively linked x-ray exposure to higher cancer death rates among radiologists.

The report described studies carried out by epidemiologists at the Johns Hopkins School of Public Health comparing the causes of death of radiologists with those of other medical specialists, using the historical cohort design described in Chapter 3. A striking and specific excess of deaths due to leukemia emerged from this important long-term investigation. Those radiologists who began their careers earlier (when there was little effort to protect either physician or patient from unnecessary radiation) had much higher rates of leukemia than their counterparts in specialties in which radiation exposure was minimal. Experimental studies with animals and the medical experience of the Japanese populations surviving the atomic bomb (followed by epidemiologists for the next forty years) have shown quite conclusively by now that ionizing radiation is leukemogenic—it can initiate leukemia.

Patients exposed to large doses of ionizing radiation also develop leukemia at a higher rate than the rest of the population. This was shown very dramatically in 1953 by the noted British epidemiologist Sir Richard Doll, who reassembled a cohort of patients with ankylosing spondylitis, a very deforming form of rheumatoid arthritis that affects mainly young men. In the United Kingdom in the 1930s and early 1940s, the treatment advocated by some rheumatologists was large doses of x-ray to the arthritic spine, to cause scarring and fusion and thus relieve some of the pain and deformity. But the bone marrow and spinal column in the path of the therapeutic x-ray contains sensitive stem cells liable to turn cancerous; and so the leukemia rate among those receiving treatment was not only very high but also correlated with the x-ray dosage. In both the atomic bomb survivors and the patients with ankylosing spondylitis the leukemia had its onset about five to ten years after the radiation was received.

Another example of iatrogenic disease related to x-ray was reported in 1989 by Canadian epidemiologists who had carried out another historical cohort study, this time on women who had been hospitalized in a tuberculosis sanatorium. There the women had received therapy whereby one of their lungs was intentionally collapsed (by adding either a lipid solution or a foreign body to the thoracic cavity). The idea was to force the lungs with the TB cavities to collapse in the hope that the cavities would then heal. These patients were examined many times using x-ray in the form of fluoroscopy on the affected side. Many years later they tended to develop breast cancer on the same side as the affected lung. That breast, of course, had received large doses of ionizing radiation. (The atomic bomb survivors also had elevated breast cancer rates compared to the Japanese population not subject to bomb blast radiation.)

The lessons learned from these investigations have informed modern therapeutic and diagnostic practice. X-rays are now deployed in the lowest possible doses, and shielding is thorough. But not all questions have been resolved. One of the continuing concerns raised by the breast cancer screening programs using mammography has been the cumulative danger from the ionizing radiation to which the breasts are exposed during the annual or biannual mammographic exam. Current thinking endorses the notion that the benefit of the procedure greatly outweighs the risk, especially since the x-ray doses have been greatly reduced with new mammogram machinery and techniques.

Adverse Drug Reactions

UNWANTED adverse reactions to drugs have received particular scrutiny from epidemiologists. One of the most interesting and unfortunate epidemics ascribable to a drug affected asthmatics in a number of different countries during the 1960s. Alarmed clinicians suddenly discovered that their young asthmatic patients were dying (death due to asthma had previously been a very rare occurrence). The epidemic had an abrupt onset

Certain countries experienced an epidemic of deaths among asthmatics during the 1960s; the epidemic curves, for ages 5 to 34, in the most severely affected countries are shown here.

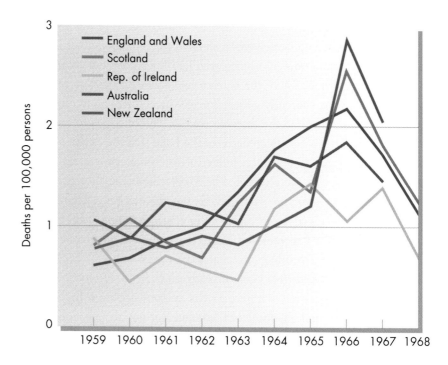

and occurred simultaneously in England, Wales, Australia, and New Zealand, but not in the United States or Canada. The graph on this page shows the epidemic curves. The rapid rise of the epidemic from 1961 to 1966 is seen in all the countries, but there was no evidence of an increase in asthma incidence, prevalence, or severity to explain the increased death rates.

The graph on the facing page depicts the introduction and use of a new medication for asthmatics first marketed in 1960; handheld, pressurized adrenergic nebulizers containing isoproterenol (called isoprenaline in the United Kingdom). The epidemic began shortly after this potent medication was introduced to relieve the air hunger that asthmatics experience. A study conducted in 1965–6 on about one hundred asthmatics who died in London and its surrounding boroughs implicated these handheld nebulizers. The study, of an unsophisticated type called a "case series," simply checked whether or not the deceased asthmatics had used the nebulizers, and indeed about 80 percent had done so. After warnings were issued by British health authorities, use of this medication declined and the epidemic waned. There was some skepticism, however, about the conclusion that the epidemic was due to the use of this new and powerful medication. After all, some countries that used the nebulizers had been spared the epidemic. If these nebulizers were the main cause of the increased deaths among asthmatics, why didn't the epidemic touch the United States and Canada, where the nebulizers were also aggressively marketed and prescribed?

The explanation turned out to be surprising. Those countries that experienced the epidemic had all marketed a particularly potent form of this medication—one five times stronger than that licensed and marketed in the United States and Canada. While this superpotent form of the nebulizer captured one-third of the market in England, two-thirds of the asthmatics who died in the case series had been using this form of the drug. Further, the mortality among asthmatics was mainly in young children who were not noted to be doing badly with their asthma prior to their deaths, which were unexpected and without warning. It was suggested that the deaths were mainly due to cardiac arrhythmias stimulated by overuse of this particularly potent form of isoproterenol. Indeed, this drug

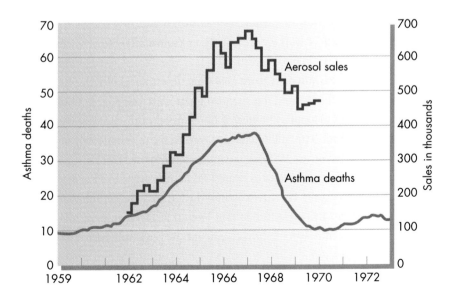

The increase in deaths among asthmatics correlated well with the widespread adoption of new handheld pressurized nebulizers containing a potent adrenergic agent designed to relieve the air hunger of asthmatics.

145

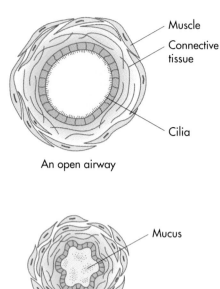

An open airway

A narrowed airway

Asthma is a reversible constriction of the airways in the lung. During an asthma attack, muscle constriction narrows the airways and they become filled with mucus, causing the symptom of air hunger so distressing to the asthmatic. The handheld nebulizers relieved the symptom but were dangerous for some patients.

had previously been used to treat persons whose heart rate was so slow that they fainted, a condition called "complete heart block," or the Adams-Stokes disease. Taking the isoproterenol in an oral form sped up the heart rate and prevented the faints, so it is clear that the drug had a powerful stimulatory effect on the heart.

Given this history, it was surprising that a second epidemic of asthma mortality continued for over a decade in New Zealand before the possible relationship of these increased deaths to the use of asthma medication was explored—but such was the case. Although the rise in mortality began in 1976, a case-control study with a primary interest in the possible association of drug use with death from asthma was not launched until the late 1980s. A group of researchers from Wellington, New Zealand, led by epidemiologist Neal Pearce and his associates, eventually carried out several case-control studies of asthma mortality that showed excess use of a particular nebulized medication not licensed in the United States. These investigations stirred much controversy, but when use of the drug was greatly reduced beginning in 1989, the asthma death rates dropped and the epidemic ended.

Epidemiology, by providing a surveillance system to monitor adverse drug effects, helps to protect the safety of our drug supply. Suspected drug reactions, which are reported routinely to drug manufacturers and the Food and Drug Administration, are analyzed and investigated; in this way, rare or delayed as well as previously unknown adverse reactions can be discovered and the risks quantified.

One well-known adverse drug reaction illustrates both the need for continuous surveillance and the requirement that beneficial claims for drugs be critically evaluated by use of the method of the randomized controlled clinical trial. The substance at issue was the female hormone diethylstilbestrol (DES). In 1949, a prestigious group of Harvard investigators advocated this synthetically created and orally ingested hormone as a remedy for miscarriage. The investigators based their recommendation on several small case series—studies that looked at the results of giving the drug to a number of pregnant women but did not examine any controls or randomize the treatment.

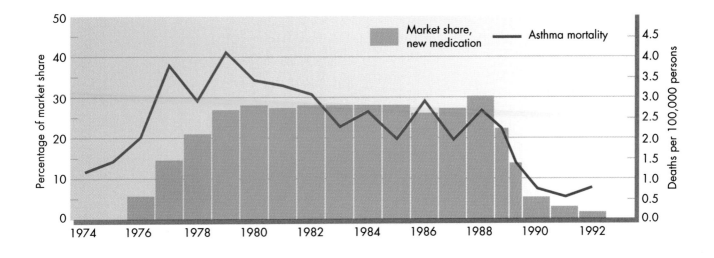

If a pregnant woman began to bleed and a miscarriage threatened, oral ingestion of DES tablets was recommended in the belief that this would reduce the chance of a subsequent miscarriage. (The embryo was simultaneously exposed to this hormone through the blood circulation that mother and fetus share.) The practice of giving pregnant women DES was widespread during the 1950s and in some communities it is estimated that during the peak years of usage as many as 15 percent of all pregnant women received it. In 1958 a study was carried out at the University of Chicago Medical Center, where pregnant women were randomized to receive either DES or an inert placebo. This randomized placebo-controlled trial showed no benefit from DES in the prevention of miscarriage, and the use of this prophylactic regimen gradually lost favor.

In 1971, however, the medical world was startled by a mini-epidemic of vaginal cancer in adolescent girls reported in the Boston area. This tumor is highly unusual in young women; in addition, those cancers associated with the Boston cluster had a distinctive microscopic appearance, being "clear-cell" adenocarcinoma.

That same year a case-control study was quickly completed by Arthur Herbst, Howard Ulfelder, and David Poskanzer. Of the eight cases of vaginal cancer in adolescent girls in the cluster, seven had been exposed

The probable cause of an epidemic of asthma deaths, which continued for over a dozen years in New Zealand, was recognized by some investigators in Wellington who carried out a series of epidemiologic studies that led to restriction of the suspected drug, Fenoterol. As the sales and use of this drug declined, so did the asthma mortality rate. This drug was never approved or marketed in the United States because the sponsoring company withdrew it from the FDA approval process for reasons the FDA cannot divulge.

One of the reasons epidemiologists were able to discover the cause of the epidemic was that the histopathology of the DES-induced tumors was so peculiar, being a clear-cell adenocarcinoma. The micrograph shows the clear cells of the glands that line the vagina as they appear when altered by the cancer.

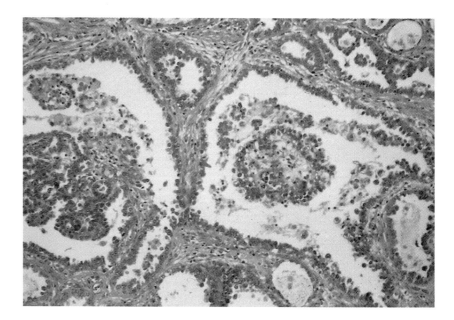

in utero to DES. None of the 32 controls—girls born in the same hospital as the cases, within a day or two—had had such exposures.

Animal experiments were initiated by experimental toxicologists, who showed that pregnant rodents given DES gave birth to female progeny who developed genital tract tumors at a much higher rate than the control animals not given DES. Thus an animal model was established, adding to the evidence that DES, by acting as a transplacental carcinogen, was the probable cause of the vaginal cancer in young women. Other evidence began to come together: a case-control study in New York State using the State Tumor Registry confirmed the study from Boston. All told, more than 600 cases of genital tract cancer were reported as a result of prenatal exposure to DES. Some deaths occurred, and drastic surgery was required for many cases with this tumor.

Not only had the DES not accomplished what it was prescribed to do, but it had also been well known as a carcinogen as far back as the early 1940s. DES was even used by some researchers to *cause* cancer in rodents so that drugs against cancer could be tested. There is no evidence that DES induced cancer in males exposed in utero (although this is still not known for certain), but it did produce anomalies of the male urogenital system. The substance still has a few justifiable medical uses: it is often administered to males to treat disseminated prostate cancer, a hormone-dependent tumor that responds favorably to DES. And DES has been used as a postcoital contraceptive in many college health services.

To illustrate the clinical significance of epidemiologic methods, note that a cohort study done in the mid-1970s in Olmstead County, Minnesota, by investigators at the Mayo Clinic did not show any cases of vaginal cancer in over 800 young women who had been exposed to DES in utero. This is not as surprising as it may first seem. Fortunately, only one in 1,000 to one in 10,000 DES-exposed women go on to develop the cancer. The cohort method is not the best way to examine such low incidence, as the negative Mayo study clearly shows. Yet the Boston case-control study answered the question of causation in a study of only 40 subjects, only 8 of them cases of the tumor and 32 of them controls.

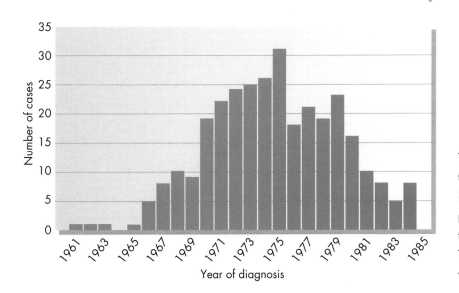

The epidemic of vaginal cancer attributed to in utero exposure to diethylstilbestrol (DES) lasted more than twenty years and peaked in 1975, about twenty years after the peak use of DES by pregnant women. The median age of the cases at diagnosis was 19 years.

A Misguided Use of Hormones

ANOTHER female hormone responsible for an epidemic of cancer was unopposed estrogen, whose use by menopausal women peaked in the mid-1970s. About two decades ago the use of this hormone replacement therapy became so popular that in some communities almost 30 percent of women had at least one course of these female hormones by the age of 65. Advertisements in the medical journals of that time and earlier suggested that administration of female hormones could reduce anxiety, relieve depression, and even help women deal with the "empty nest syndrome."

While the drug manufacturer's advertisements did not suggest so, many women also believed that these hormones would prevent the wrinkling of skin that accompanies aging. A best-selling book entitled *Feminine Forever* advocated that *all* women should take such hormones, making the argument that menopause was not part of natural aging but rather a medical disorder treatable by hormone replacement. A famous endocrinologist wrote the foreword to the book, which now seems ludicrous in its zealotry:

> Like a gallant knight [the author of *Feminine Forever*] has come to rescue his fair lady not at the time of her bloom and flowering but in her dispairing years; at a time of life when the preservation and prolongation of her femaleness are so paramount. . . . By throwing down his gauntlet, he challenges the reluctant physician to follow him in providing the hormones that may allow for a smoother transition to the menopausal years ahead. Woman will be emancipated only when the shackles of hormonal deprivation are loosed.

Epidemiologists, however, noted an increase in the incidence and mortality from uterine cancer during the period that the estrogen replacement therapy became popular and widely used in the United States. Since hysterectomy rates were rising at the same time, the uterine cancer rate was actually *under*estimated in official statistics, because the denomina-

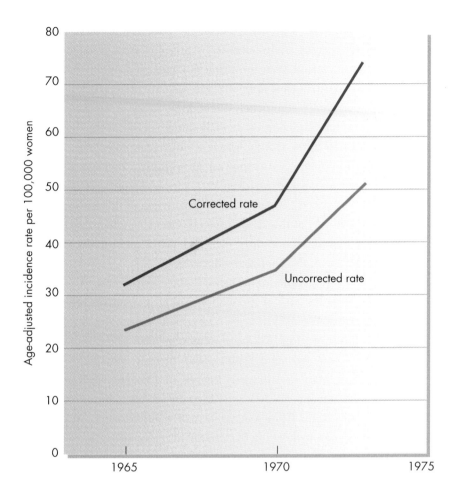

The graph shows the incidence rate over time for cancer of the uterus both taking into account the underlying hysterectomy rate in the population and ignoring it. When it is ignored, the incidence rate appears lower than it actually is because included in the population at risk (the denominator) are women who are really not at risk of this cancer since their uterus has been removed. The corrected rate is higher, although the slope and contour of the two rates are similar.

tor for the rate included hysterectomized women (without a uterus, none of them was at risk for the tumor).

More than ten case-control studies and several cohort investigations showed an association of uterine cancer with hormone replacement therapy. The risk increased as the duration of the therapy increased. Even if a woman used hormones for only a few years, her risk of uterine cancer was several times greater than that of a nonuser; but if she used the hormones for more than five years, her risk climbed to as much as fifteen times that of a nonuser. The most common form of hormone replacement therapy twenty years ago was the administration by pill of estrone, a female estrogenic hormone harvested from the urine of pregnant mares—hence the trade name Premarin. (This hormone was given "unopposed," that is, without a concomitantly administered female hormone of the progestogen type. Currently the hormone is usually given simultaneously with a progestogen for part of the month, which seems to counteract the carcinogenic effect of the unopposed estrogen.) As warnings went out about the dangers of using unopposed estrogen as a supplemental or replacement therapy, its use declined—and so did the incidence of the associated tumor. During the height of this drug-induced cancer "epidemic," however, it is estimated that about one-third of the uterine cancer cases could be attributed to the use of the unopposed hormone.

At present the popularity of hormone replacement therapy has undergone a renaissance because of the evidence that its use can prevent osteoporosis ("bone softening") in women after menopause; thus it may prevent hip fractures in elderly women. There is also some increasingly persuasive data that hormone replacement therapy may help prevent heart attacks. But there are still many unanswered questions about proper dose, length of treatment needed, possible cancer risks, and the value of the added progestogen. Epidemiologists will contribute to the ongoing search for knowledge by keeping the treatment under surveillance and by both urging and performing the needed randomized controlled studies and nonexperimental (cohort and case-control) investigations.

An Epidemic from an Over-the-Counter Drug

OVER-the-counter drugs, for which no prescription is needed, can also cause epidemics. Although these are not strictly speaking iatrogenic (physician-induced), epidemiological expertise is a key to investigating illness arising from self-medication, just as from prescribed medication. One fairly recent epidemic of a completely new disease occurred in the United States and several other countries as the result of a contaminated food supplement.

An eosinophil is a white blood cell that functions as part of the immune system. Recognized by its double-lobed nucleus, an eosinophil contains numerous granules from which substances toxic to foreign cells may be released. The particular targets of eosinophils are parasitic worms and allergens.

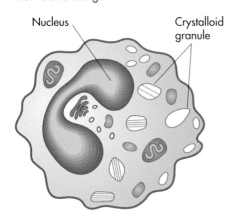

Nucleus

Crystalloid granule

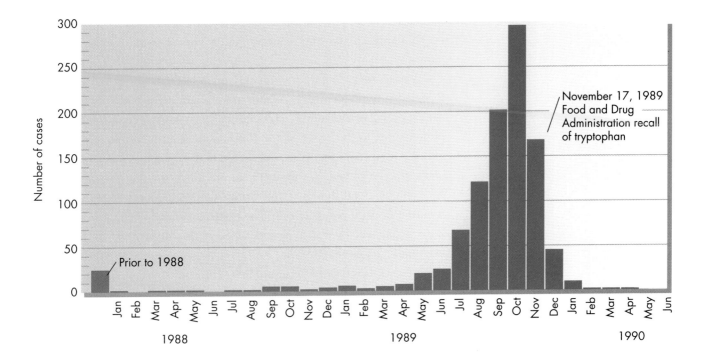

The epidemic curve for the eosinophilia myalgia syndrome shows the abrupt rise of the epidemic, which peaked in October 1989. This pattern is typical of "common source" outbreaks, for which a single cause or exposure is responsible.

In 1989 several physicians in New Mexico were consulted by patients who presented a very strange disorder. They complained of extremely severe muscle aches, fatigue, skin rashes, and neurologic symptoms. When blood counts were performed, they showed a striking *eosinophilia*—the term used for an increase in the number of eosinophils circulating in the blood. This blood cell is often "high" in such diseases as trichinosis, certain severe allergies, and a few other, rare illnesses. Most of the initial patients seen in New Mexico were young or middle-aged women; moreover, the epidemic disease had a sudden onset, clustering in time (late 1989) and place (New Mexico).

The treating physicians ruled out trichinosis and obtained a detailed history of drugs taken by the patients, since drug reactions will occasionally cause eosinophil counts to rise. They discovered that all of the initial cases had patronized "natural" food stores, where they obtained a food supplement containing the amino acid L-tryptophan. This food supplement was being touted for relief of insomnia and depression, and the women took it in large amounts, becoming ill shortly after starting to use it. This seemed the only common thread or exposure linking the first cases.

A case-control study was quickly organized. All 12 of the cases had ingested L-tryptophan pills, mainly purchased at specialty nutrition food stores; only 2 of 22 controls ingested the same substance during the same period prior to the onset of the illness experienced by the cases. With only 34 subjects in the study, the source of the epidemic was to all intents and purposes solved. A warning went out about the dangers of ingesting L-tryptophan, and the Food and Drug Administration arranged to have it removed from all points of sale. The epidemic ended once these measures were taken, but over a thousand cases of this mysterious disease were eventually reported. The disease, given the name *eosinophilia myalgia syndrome (EMS)*, is still being studied. The epidemic was finally traced to the product of a single Japanese manufacturer, who by changing the manufacturing process for the substance had somehow introduced one or more toxic contaminants. Their precise chemical structures are still not known for certain.

One of the authors of this volume (Paul Stolley) saw one of the earliest cases of EMS in his internal medicine practice. He had no way of realizing there was more than a single case, or that clusters were being seen in other localities. Only when he read about the New Mexico cluster did he recognize that he had seen one of the very earliest cases in an epidemic. This is a vivid illustration of the importance of communicating information about suspected new diseases, which are often so rare that a single practitioner may see only one or two, unaware that an epidemic is in progress. (The early case seen, queried about L-tryptophan use, confirmed this and located her empty bottles. She had indeed been taking the substance shipped by the implicated manufacturer.)

Failures of quality control analogous to the cause of EMS can occur at any time—and they are by no means limited to over-the-counter pharmaceuticals. One telling example will suffice here. The national campaign to immunize the U.S. population against polio in 1956 was nearly wrecked because of a contaminated lot of the Salk vaccine. Not properly processed, it harbored live virus. This bad lot (produced by the Cutter

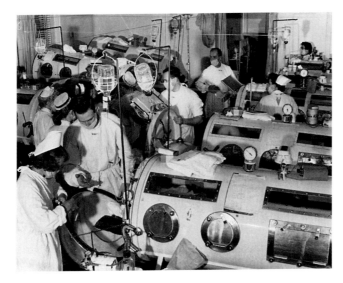

Polio could damage the nervous control of the diaphragm, leading to trouble breathing. The "iron lung" was developed to help assist the breathing of polio victims. There were over 20,000 cases annually of paralytic polio in the years before the national campaign to vaccinate the children of the United States using the newly invented Salk vaccine.

Company) actually caused over one hundred cases of the disease it was designed to prevent. A very rapid and detailed investigation quickly identified the fact that a single bad lot of vaccine was responsible; the rest of the vaccine supply was safe. This allowed the halted vaccination campaign to again proceed, and the successful campaign cut the number of cases from 21,000 to less tha 100 between the years 1952 and 1964.

A Pharmaceutical Tragedy

DRUGSTORES and pharmacies sell more than just prescribed medications and home remedies. One of the most tragic and puzzling epidemics caused by an over-the-counter product occurred in France in 1972 but was described for the first time ten years later in *The Lancet*. According to French law, the facts about this epidemic had to be concealed for a decade until the litigation concerning the epidemic had ended.

The epidemic came to notice when a number of infants were referred to the pediatric neurology service of a large Paris teaching hospital. These infants had developed a bizarre and previously undescribed neurologic illness accompanied by a remarkably severe rash in the diaper area, on the neck, or both. The infants first became excitable and irritable and appeared to be in pain; as the days progressed and the illness worsened, they showed signs of severe brain damage, with coma and death ensuing. When the epidemic ended, 34 infants had died, including one pair of twins. Several had improved while in the hospital, only to be sent home, where they worsened and died.

The epidemic began in the month of April 1972 and ended about September of the same year, affecting about 120 infants. The classic technique of locating each case on a map (spot-mapping) was used, and the

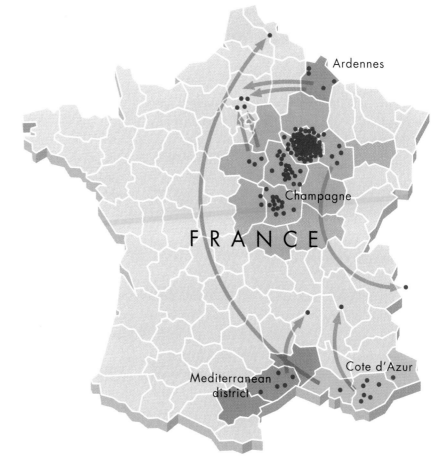

The epidemic of a new and strange neurological illness in France had a distinct geographic distribution on a spot map. It later turned out that this geographical pattern could be explained by the delivery of contaminated baby powder to large chain drugstores by trucks from the factory. The rare cases outside the area were the result of a traveler buying the powder while passing through the area where the contaminated product had been delivered.

epidemic was seen to be concentrated in the Ardennes and Côte d'Azur regions of France. And yet no affected infant had contact with any other except in a case of twins; indeed, the parents of the victims did not know each other. Person-to-person transmission was therefore deemed unlikely. Attempts to isolate or culture a transmissible infectious agent were fruitless, and epidemiologists visiting the homes of the victims found only one "exposure" common to the affected infants. The parents had all used the same baby powder, one of the most popular in France, called BéBé.

Although this seemed a slim lead, bottles of the powder were sampled from the shelves of stores in Paris, and chemical analysis revealed that the contents were exactly as listed: talc and fragrance. Thus the search for a toxic contaminant at first seemed to come to a dead end. The epidemic continued and new cases appeared. Again the investigation revealed the only common exposure to be BéBé. This time the investigators analyzed the *actual bottles used by the mothers* on the affected infants. Now the chemists found (in addition to the talc and fragrance) the chemical hexachlorophene at over 6 percent concentration by weight.

Hexachlorophene was then used as an antibacterial agent in cosmetics and soaps. Its toxic properties when ingested are well known because accidental poisonings have occurred when people swallowed unlabeled portions of the white milky hexachlorophene emulsion (a liquid soap) marketed around the world as Phisohex, thinking it was an antacid or milk of magnesia. The signs and symptoms of the poisoning were primarily neurologic, the hexachlorophene seeking out fatty tissues such as the white matter of the brain and destroying brain tissues by disrupting metabolism. These adult oral poisonings presented a clinical picture much like that seen in the French infants. But the infants had been poisoned percutaneously—through the skin! The hexachlorophene in high concentration had irritated and damaged the babies' skin, producing the terrible rash in the diaper area or the neck (a favorite place for French mothers to powder their infants). The broken skin was no longer a barrier to absorption of the hexachlorophene, which could now enter the bloodstream and deposit in the fatty brain tissue, killing the infants or seriously damaging their nervous systems.

The bottles of the powder sampled from Paris stores were innocent, as the contaminated lot of bottles was distributed only in large chain drugstores of the Ardennes and Côte d'Azur. That explained the geographic distribution of the disease. When the bottles actually used on sick infants were analyzed, the contamination was identified correctly and all bottles seized and removed from store shelves; but it was late in the epidemic. Almost all had been sold.

The contaminated lot was produced in a factory where several products were made, depending on the day of the week and the demand. One of the products contained hexachlorophene. A barrel of white hexachlorophene powder was confused with the similar-appearing white talc used in the baby powder during one production lot. About 3,000 bottles were mixed containing dangerous 6-percent hexachlorophene.

During the litigation initiated by the relatives of the dead infants, videotapes were shown in court of infant baboons who were powdered and diapered using the contaminated powder in exactly the same manner as had been the human infants. One of us (Paul Stolley) had the opportunity to view these films, and watched as, day by day, the baboons were examined. The pathetic deterioration of their neurologic condition was clear and ghastly to behold. The experience for the parents of the affected infants must have been horrific.

When these accidents happen and produce disease, it is the responsibility of the epidemiologist to try to track down the problem as quickly as possible and prevent further cases. This epidemic was skillfully investigated and solved by Dr. Gilbert Martin-Bouyer and his associates, working for the French government agency called INSERM. He subsequently helped to solve an even more deadly and bizarre poisoning that took place in Vietnam after the war ended—again through the agency of baby powder.

A peculiar disease of infants began suddenly in August 1981 in Ho Chi Minh City (formerly called Saigon). The infants, ranging in age from fifteen days to three months, began to bruise easily and then to bleed into the gut. Eventually 741 infants developed the illness, and 177 died from hemorrhage before the epidemic ended. All efforts to find an infectious agent or to link the disease to person-to-person transmission failed. When

Dr. Martin-Bouyer was called to Vietnam as a consultant, his experience with the BéBé epidemic led him to speculate whether a toxic substance might have been applied to the infants' skin. The mothers in a sample of cases were interviewed using a questionnaire, and again the one thing common to all cases was the use of baby talcum powder (an uncommon practice in Vietnam at that time). It finally turned out that the rat poison coumadin (Warfarin), which interferes with blood clotting, had been added to the baby powder. Coumadin was identified in the bulk stock of the manufacturer, although the source of the contamination and the reasons for it were never clearly unraveled.

Vietnam's economy was in such poor shape that baby powder, like other consumer items, was often made in apartments or "fly-by-night" factories. The bottles in which the powder was sold had no factory identification and were of varied shapes, sizes, and markings. Was the coumadin put in the powder to deliberately poison and kill these babies? This is very unlikely, as no cases of percutaneous poisoning of infants with coumadin had ever been reported. Possible, but unproved, is the theory that it was added as an inexpensive fragrance—coumadin powder has a weak perfumelike scent. Whatever the motivation, the anticoagulant coumadin was absorbed into the infants' bloodstreams just like the hexachlorophene, and it caused the hemorrhage and eventual death of hundreds of infants until warnings could be put out by appropriate health authorities. Once the cause was known, moreover, new cases could be treated successfully by giving vitamin K, which directly counteracts the anticoagulant effect of the coumadin. A study carried out on infant baboons, which replicated the syndrome by applying the powder to the baboon's shaved skin, proved that coumadin could be absorbed through the skin.

Ensuring a Safe Drug Supply

MOST advanced industrial nations have a government regulatory authority whose mandate is to ensure the safety and efficacy of the drug supply, whether prescription or over-the-counter. These agencies usually are given the job of conducting surveillance over new pharmaceuticals to detect adverse drug reactions and review the evidence put forth for the manufacturer's or sponsor's claims for the drug. For example, in the case of a new antihypertensive drug, they would want to know, does the compound really lower blood pressure? If it does, does this reduce the dangerous consequences of hypertension? And what are the compound's side effects?

The continuing surveillance of drugs that have been put on the market is essential if rare and delayed reactions are ever to be reliably detected. Consider how many people have to have taken a drug if a very rare but serious reaction—it occurs in only one out of 100,000 uses—is to be detected. The often fatal aplastic anemia caused by the antibiotic chloramphenicol is a good example that took some years to be detected: this rare but serious dose-related reaction occurs in perhaps one out of 60,000 users. Since there is often a safer substitute drug, even this low risk is seldom worth running. For this reason, chloramphenicol prescriptions are usually limited to severe infections for which no alternative drug is available.

The laws governing drug approval evolved slowly and usually in response to catastrophes—drug-caused epidemics like those in the table on the facing page. The 1938 Food and Drug Act established tougher safety and quality control manufacturing standards as a direct response to the deaths of more than one hundred children who died from ingesting a pediatric form of a sulfonamide antibiotic that had been dissolved in ethylene glycol (antifreeze) by the manufacturer. The elixir was never tested in animals, and the solution was highly toxic.

Still, drugs did not have to be proven efficacious—a manufacturer did not legally have to prove its claims for the drug—until the Food and Drug Act was amended in 1962. This so-called Kefauver amendment (named after Senator Estes Kefauver, who proposed it and pushed its congressional approval, strengthening the law in several ways) was possible because of the thalidomide disaster.

Thalidomide was a hypnotic (a drug that induces sleep), promoted as being particularly safe for pregnant women although there was no evidence to support this unwarranted claim. As a result, many fetuses were

Some Important Epidemics Caused by Drug Therapies

Year	
1884	Nearly 200 factory workers in Bremen, Germany, who received smallpox vaccine contaminated with human sera, developed hepatitis.
1937	Over 100 persons, mainly children, died in the United States after ingesting elixir sulfanilamide, which had been manufactured using the solvent, diethylene glycol.
1940–55	Thousands of babies blinded from retrolental fibroplasia, a disease of the retinal vasculature, as a result of the high oxygen concentrations used to treat premature infants.
1944	Hundreds of persons in North and South America developed hepatitis after receiving a yellow fever vaccine contaminated with human sera.
1955	Over 100 cases of paralytic poliomyelitis occurred in children in the United States after they received a certain lot of Salk polio vaccine produced by Cutter Laboratories. Live polio virus was present in the vaccine as an effect of the failure to inactivate the virus completely.
1959–62	About 500 infants in Germany and over 1,000 others elsewhere were born with phocomelia due to maternal use of the hypnotic thalidomide.
1960–67	An estimated several thousand excess deaths among asthmatics in the United Kingdom, New Zealand, and Australia were thought to be due to use of pressurized nebulizers containing an adrenergic agent (isoproterenol).
1962	A drug used in Europe and the United States to lower serum cholesterol, MER-29, was found to cause cataracts in some of the recipients.
1971–80	Over 380 cases of adenocarcinoma of the vagina in young women in the United States were reported to a central registry in Boston. Ninety percent had a history of in utero exposure to diethylstilbestrol.

exposed to the drug in utero, where it unfortunately produced a rather unique congenital anomaly called phocomelia. Phocomelia designates the absence of all or part of a limb. Babies born with this condition are severely disabled, usually requiring prosthetic devices. Some have to learn to write with their feet rather than their absent hands. The limb develop-

Those individuals who developed phocomelia from exposure to thalidomide in utero often made remarkable adjustments to their disabilities. These photographs show how the absence of arms was compensated for by remarkable use of the lower limbs.

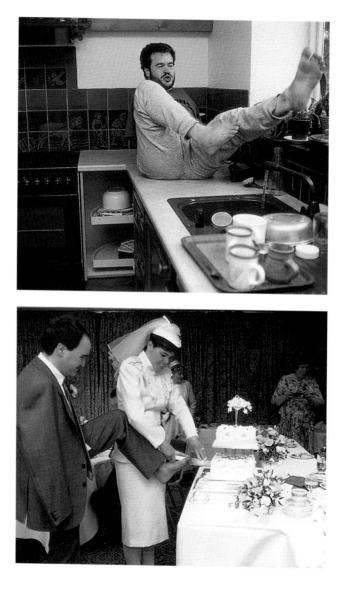

ment of the embryo is somehow interfered with by thalidomide, and hundreds of children were born in Europe with this terrible disability.

There were very few cases in the United States, however, because no license to market the drug was approved. The FDA's review officer, Dr. Florence Kelsey, asked for more toxicological information, believing the drug to have been inadequately studied. But it was approved for use in most of Europe, and that is where the first cases occurred. Dr. W. Lenz of (then) West Germany connected the sudden appearance of this birth defect with thalidomide use, and later epidemiological studies confirmed his initial observations. Any dispute about the role of thalidomide as a cause of this birth defect was put to rest by the swiftness with which the epidemic ended after the drug was banned and removed from the market.

The balance between ensuring safety and speeding effective new drugs to market is often hard to achieve, and there is still controversy about these issues. But the United States now has much safer and more effective drugs available than was the case before the Food and Drug Act was strengthened. Epidemiological surveillance of drugs continues to be an important safeguard for doctors and patients, offering another example of the practical application of epidemiological methods to real health problems.

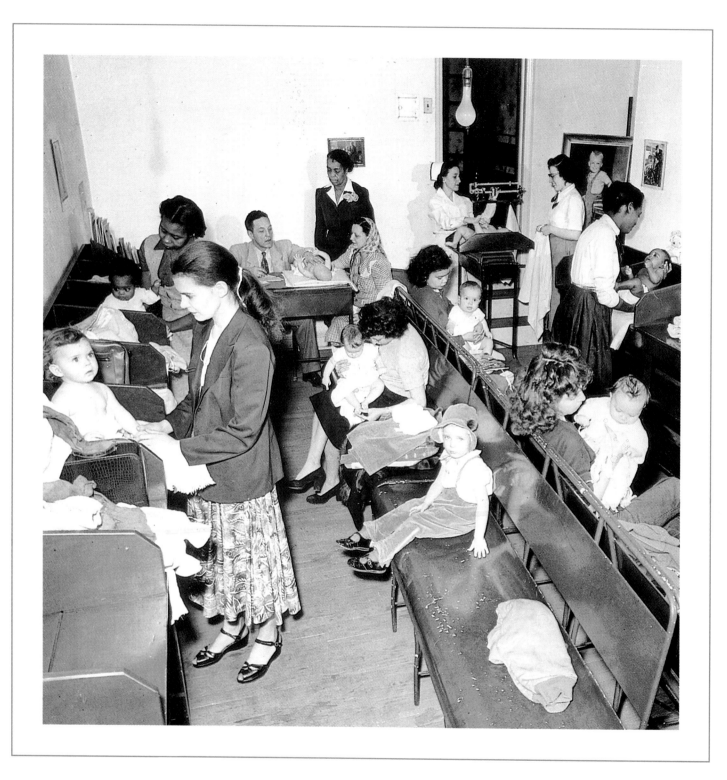

7

Screening Populations: Costs, Risks, and Benefits

PARENTS AND children await their turn to see the doctor in a child-care clinic of the 1950s. Screening for disease in its early stages is one function of such clinics. The question for epidemiologists is, Do screening tests actually prolong life?

A goal of modern medicine is to seek out people who are in the early stages of a disease so that they may be treated and the disease's progression brought to a halt. Sometimes it is even possible to find healthy people who are at risk of a disease so that its occurrence may be completely prevented. Screening tests are relatively simple procedures that can be performed on a large group of people and that detect individuals in the early stages of disease or at risk of disease. Many screening tests are hardly recognized as such, so thoroughly have they been incorporated into routine checkups, well-baby visits, prenatal care, and other clinical encounters. Weight and blood pressure measurements are examples of the simplest and most common screening procedures; they are informative in a great variety of individuals and conditions, cheap, easy, and noninvasive—simple to incorporate into an office setting. The physical or checkup is itself a screening procedure, aimed at identifying problems and intervening to prevent the worsening of any adverse condition or to correct it (with vitamin supplements, vaccinations, blood pressure medication, eyeglasses, and so on).

Many widely used screening procedures are highly specific tests for particular illnesses. The tuberculosis tine test, measurement of cholesterol, mammography, and the Pap test are examples of common medical procedures carried out routinely on symptom-free people. With the development of each new screening procedure, there are a variety of questions to be answered before the procedure can be placed into widespread use. Does the test identify people with the disease accurately enough to be used at all? Is it more accurate or more beneficial for certain segments of the population—particular age groups, for example? Does the use of a given screening test result in better health for a population? That is, is adequate treatment available to those diagnosed with the disease? Can finding the disease and subsequent treatment prevent the disease's more serious consequences? These are questions that epidemiologists can make disciplined attempts to resolve, using the methods that serve them well elsewhere, including controlled studies and statistical analyses of data describing a population. The information gathered by epidemiologists is taken into account by professional organizations, insurers, the

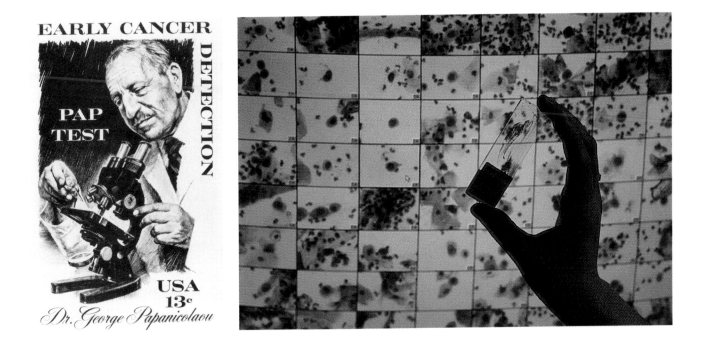

government, and others who formulate recommendations for how to use a test—when to give the test and to whom.

Screening tests were first used to prevent the spread of communicable diseases such as tuberculosis or syphilis. Tests like the tine test and chest x-ray for tuberculosis and the Wassermann blood test for syphilis, introduced early in this century, were meant to prevent the transmission of disease by identifying infected people and limiting their activities. Screening before employment kept tuberculosis-infected people from unknowingly spreading their illness in the workplace, while the Wassermann test was intended to preclude the spread of syphilis to one's future spouse. Screening tests continue to be useful in the control of infectious disease, most notably in today's meticulous screening of donated blood products, which is designed to prevent the transmission of HIV through the blood supply. As is true of blood screening for HIV, infectious disease screening often aims first at prevention—not for the screened individual, but for his or her other contacts.

This U.S. postal stamp (left) honors Dr. George Papanicolaou, the developer of the "Pap test" used to screen for early signs of cervical cancer. A specimen taken from the cervix is placed on a glass slide and stained, then photographed under a microscope so that it can be examined for cancerous cells. The array of stains in the photograph to the right are all from pap smears.

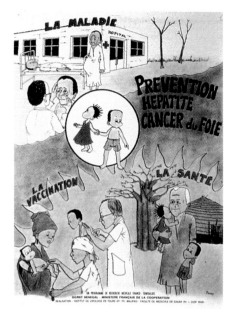

Vaccination campaigns are one example of modern attempts at preventing disease.

Aside from the control of infectious disease, screening has assumed greater importance in recent decades in the control and prevention of noninfectious diseases, such as heart disease and cancer. Well into the nineteenth century, many people even in industrialized countries lived their whole lives without ever seeing a doctor, even when they could afford the doctor's fees, or sent for a doctor only when illness or injury struck (as is still often true outside the industrialized world). Medical practitioners saw their main task as the treatment and cure of illness. Our rapid increase in scientific knowledge and understanding of disease processes has enabled medicine to begin addressing the causes of illness, with the object both to cure and prevent disease. With the introduction at the turn of the century of simple preventive measures such as vitamin supplements and vaccines, physicians and nurses began seeing themselves as advocates and agents of prevention, and their patients, too, began to see the value of regular physical exams. Today, apparently healthy people visit health care professionals with the purpose of discovering underlying diseases or forestalling illness that might occur in the future.

One result of this shift in attitude is an increased use of screening procedures in all aspects of medical care and as a public health activity. Screening takes place not only in the doctor's office but also in the community—in the mall, in schools, sometimes in the workplace. Where, when, to whom, and how often to give a screening test are the subjects of recommendations made by professional organizations and advocacy groups like the American Cancer Society; it is then up to the individual doctor to follow the recommendations or an advocacy group to organize a community screening effort. Sometimes the government mandates screening tests—for schoolchildren or military personnel, for example. Employers and unions may also take the initiative in promoting the well-being of their employees by offering some screening tests on the work site.

The scientific data gathered in epidemiologic studies is an important element in the decision making about how to use a screening test, although it is not the only element. As a tool in the fight against breast cancer, the case of mammography offers us an excellent opportunity to examine how a screening test is evaluated according to epidemiologic principles.

What is the Value of a Screening Test? The Case of Mammography

MAMMOGRAPHY provides an example of a widely used and well-studied screening procedure that may detect disease at its early stages, opening the door to successful intervention. For the past several decades health educators have encouraged women to see their doctors for regular breast exams, to examine their own breasts every month, and to undergo mammography for the detection of growths too small to be detected by clinical or self-examination.

A mammogram is an x-ray of the breast. It can show variations in breast tissue density indicating the presence of lesions or masses that may be cancerous. When a radiologist observes a positive mammogram (that is, one showing abnormal tissue), he or she refers the patient for biopsy of the tissue (surgical sampling and a pathologist's review) to determine whether disease is present. Positive mammograms do not always

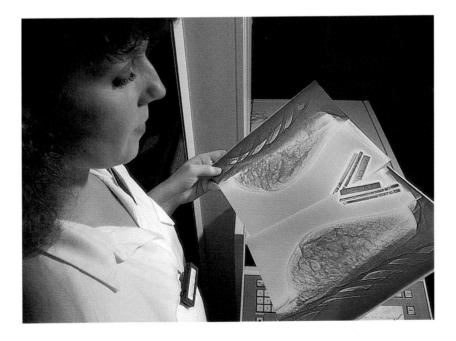

A radiologist examines a mammogram to determine whether the breast has a suspicous pattern that requires further investigation.

indicate the presence of cancer; sometimes an image that appears abnormal in the x-ray is found to be normal on biopsy. Such false positives cause great worry and inconvenience for patients, of course, as well as incurring the time and expense of further procedures.

Compensating for the various costs of false positives is the benefit derived from the detection of true positives who might not be identified otherwise. The physician's or patient's examination of the breast to detect dense or lumpy tissue can feel growths only of a certain size. A clinical exam may miss small lumps or areas of tissue density that a mammogram might detect. If mammography can detect cancers that might otherwise go undiagnosed, the procedure might lead to earlier and more successful treatment—a clear gain for the patient. When deciding whether to recommend that screening be carried out routinely in clinical practice or in the community, epidemiologists need to consider a test's ability to correctly classify people with and without the condition. Before returning again to mammography, we examine more closely how epidemiologists evaluate the accuracy of screening tests in general.

Sensitivity, Specificity, and Predictive Value

AN ideal screening test would show up positive every time the patient *had* the disease, and negative every time the patient *didn't* have the disease. All the positive tests would be *true positives,* all the negative tests would be *true negatives.* There are many reasons, however, why no screening test is ideal. Errors in reading an x-ray, handling a specimen, running a procedure, or preparing equipment can all produce incorrect test results. Errors are inevitable, but one can compensate for them by repeating the test several times. More important than these errors is the reality that most health conditions are not dichotomous, yes/no conditions, but lie along a continuum. A fracture can be so big that it can be easily diagnosed by the naked eye, or so small that several x-rays do not show it. Moreover, random variation in a condition can result in incorrect test results for those with conditions that are borderline. A patient with borderline hypertension, for example, might be screened on a day when his or her blood pressure is at a high or low fluctuation; that individual would then be classified as having high or normal blood pressure, respectively. In the early stages of a disease, all characteristics may not yet be apparent, and a test, therefore, may not detect the presence of early disease.

The concepts *sensitivity* and *specificity* provide a way to quantify a screening test's ability to detect the presence or absence of a disease. Sensitivity measures the proportion of people with a condition who are correctly classified by the test as having the condition.

$$\text{Sensitivity} = \frac{\substack{\text{number of people who test positive} \\ \text{(and truly have the condition)}}}{\substack{\text{number of people tested who} \\ \text{actually } \textit{have} \text{ the condition}}} \times 100$$

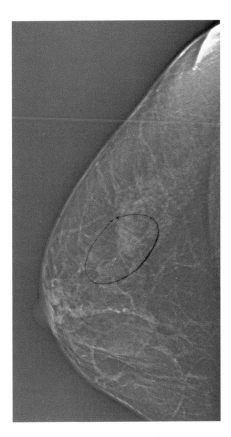

Specificity measures the proportion of people without the condition who are correctly classified by the test as not having the condition.

$$\text{Specificity} = \frac{\substack{\text{number of people who test negative} \\ \text{(and do not have the condition)}}}{\substack{\text{number of people tested who actually} \\ \text{do } \textit{not} \text{ have the condition}}} \times 100$$

The circle surrounds an area of suspected malignant tissue revealed in a mammogram. A trained radiologist can distinguish healthy tissue suspected of being cancerous.

To collect data regarding sensitivity and specificity, epidemiologists must screen a representative group of people and then assess their true disease status by some means other than the screening test. This sometimes presents its own set of logistical problems; one cannot, for example, conduct biopsies on women whose mammograms are negative. One must instead follow a group of women to observe the number of cancers occurring in the group that tested negative. This approach was taken in Canada in the National Breast Screening Study; the researchers gave mammograms to 44,718 women in 15 participating centers in the 1980s.

In the first screening, 3,067 women were found to have positive mammograms and were referred for further tests. After completing the tests, the researchers were able to calculate the number of true and false positives, noted in the cells of the table on the next page as 226 and 2,841

Results of the National Breast Screening Study

	Cancer	No cancer	
Positive mammogram	226	2,841	3,067
Negative mammogram	76	41,575	41,651
	302	44,416	44,718

women, respectively. They also collected data on women who had negative mammograms and yet were diagnosed with cancer in the next 12 months (76 women). The researchers could then derive both sensitivity and specificity from a two-by-two contingency table that compares the results of the mammograms with the "true" results, as explained in the box on the facing page. The sensitivity and specificity turned out to be 75 percent and 94 percent, respectively.

Estimates from other studies of the sensitivity of mammograms range from 71 to 78 percent (that is, 71 to 78 percent of the women tested who have breast cancer have positive mammograms). The sensitivity varies by the size of the lesion and the age of the patient. Sensitivity is higher in women over 50 (over 80 percent) and lower in women under 50 (about 60 percent). These data suggest that mammograms by themselves can miss some cases of breast cancer.

When a test is very *sensitive,* it picks up everyone screened who has the disease; but it may also pick up people who do not have the disease (false positives). Such a test may be useful for preventing the spread of infectious diseases, since it is essential to find all cases to prevent transmission. Yet high sensitivity and a high number of false positives bring a variety of costs—the anxiety of patients who, having tested positive, do not have the disease, and the time and financial liability of following up those patients, who are actually healthy. For diseases that carry terminal prognoses and severe social stigmas, like HIV infection, it is unacceptable to allow any false positives—a false positive may have terrible repercussions for a patient's insurance coverage, job security, housing, social relationships, and emotional well-being.

Characteristics of a Screening Test

Various measures have been developed to characterize screening tests, but all can be easily derived from a simple two-by-two contingency table. The table entries give the number of cases classified according to test results and actual disease status; the tests are either positive or negative and the people tested may either have the disease or not (disease status positive or negative).

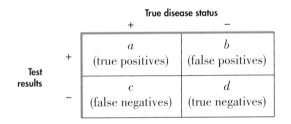

The measures of sensitivity and specificity compare true positives or true negatives, respectively, to the number of people who truly have the disease (sensitivity) or do not have the disease (specificity). It is a simple matter to plug in the values from the National Breast Screening Study to calculate these measures:

$$\text{Sensitivity} = \frac{a}{a+c} \times 100$$

$$= \frac{226}{302} \times 100 = 74.8 \text{ percent}$$

$$\text{Specificity} = \frac{d}{b+d} \times 100$$

$$= \frac{41,575}{44,416} \times 100 = 93.6 \text{ percent}$$

The measures of positive and negative predictive value compare the number of true positives and true negatives, respectively, to the number of people who tested positive (in the case of positive predictive value) or negative (in the case of negative predictive value). Plugging in the values from the breast screening study, we obtain:

$$\text{Positive predictive value} = \frac{a}{a+b} \times 100$$

$$= \frac{226}{3,067} \times 100 = 7 \text{ percent}$$

$$\text{Negative predictive value} = \frac{d}{c+d} \times 100$$

$$= \frac{41,575}{41,651} \times 100 = 99.8 \text{ percent}$$

Of the women who test positive, only 7 percent will truly have cancer; the rest will undergo unnecessary biopsy and worry. Of the women who test negative, a very small percentage (0.2 percent) will have cancer that may go undetected.

When a test is very *specific*, all of the people who are truly free of disease will test negative, but the group testing negative will probably also include some people who have the disease (false negatives). Since the goal of screening is to identify people with a given disease or condition, it is naturally desirable to keep the number of false negatives to a minimum.

A screening test may also be judged by its predictive value. The predictive value of a positive test is the proportion of people testing positive who truly have the disease.

$$\text{Positive predictive value} = \frac{\text{true positives}}{\text{all those who test positive}} \times 100$$

The predictive value of a negative test is, similarly, the proportion of people testing negative who are truly free of disease.

$$\text{Negative predictive value} = \frac{\text{true negatives}}{\text{all those who test negative}} \times 100$$

The National Breast Screening Study had found 226 true positives out of a total of 3,067 positive test results, for a positive predictive value of 7 percent. This low value means that for every true positive test result, more than a dozen women will experience the worry and possible inconvenience of a false positive.

The predictive value of a test increases with the prevalence of the condition in a given population. When a condition is more prevalent, there will be more true positives, yet the specificity—the number of false negatives—will remain the same. A higher ratio of true positives to false positives produces a higher predictive value.

The tables on the facing page illustrate how the predictive value of a disease increases as its prevalence rises from 1 to 50 percent. Assuming that sensitivity remains fixed at 90 percent and specificity at 95 percent, predictive value increases from 15.2 percent to 48.9 percent to 94.7 percent as prevalence increases from 1 to 5 to 50 percent. A screening test will more successfully predict whether or not a person has a disease when

Contingency Tables for (from left to right) Prevalences of 1, 5, and 50 Percent

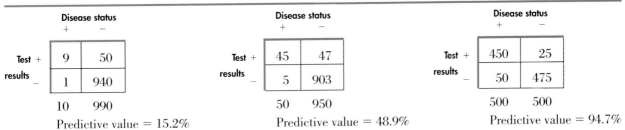

	Disease status +	Disease status −
Test +	9	50
results −	1	940
	10	990

Predictive value = 15.2%

	Disease status +	Disease status −
Test +	45	47
results −	5	903
	50	950

Predictive value = 48.9%

	Disease status +	Disease status −
Test +	450	25
results −	50	475
	500	500

Predictive value = 94.7%

the disease is more common i.e., has a higher prevalance rate. For this reason, many screening programs are designed to target groups of people in which the disease is highly prevalent and the predictive value high. It seems intuitively reasonable to screen for a condition among people who are likely to have the condition, that is, to screen for sickle-cell anemia among African Americans, or for glaucoma among the elderly. Focusing the efforts of a community-screening program on a target population can help justify the program's cost because less money is spent on screening people without the condition.

Do Mammograms Save Lives?

SENSITIVITY, specificity, and predictive value are not the only criteria for a screening test. To be of value to the patient (not just to the research scientist), any screening must—if positive—be associated with the possibility of treatment that offers hope. After identifying cases it is necessary to follow up with treatments that lead to the prevention of either the disease or its adverse effects. In the case of breast cancer, the question is whether mammography leads to earlier diagnosis of breast cancer and therefore to more effective treatment and increased survival rates. One of the tenets of preventive medicine is that it is better to treat a disease in its early stages. This seems intuitively reasonable; certainly cancer, when diagnosed very late, is untreatable. Does earlier detection of breast cancer improve the prospects for survival? What types of data do we need to show this?

We have two sources of data concerning breast cancer in the general population: data about newly diagnosed cases of breast cancer, and data about deaths caused by breast cancer. For certain conditions, the goal of screening is prevention, but we don't expect mammographic screening to result in a decrease in the number of breast cancer cases; in this situation screening is a means of finding *earlier* cases. Institution of a screening procedure like mammography may, indeed, reveal previously undetected cases and produce an apparent rise in the incidence of the disease. If the screening program continues and women continue to receive earlier diagnoses, this initial rise may show up as an artificial and temporary increase in incidence. After the change in detection is established as routine, incidence rates should again reflect usual patterns of disease occurrence.

We hope that screening will result in longer life expectancy for women diagnosed with breast cancer. But what if, by diagnosing women in earlier stages of disease, we merely lengthen the period between diagnosis and death, artificially increasing our measure of survival without truly improving life expectancy? To rule out this potential distortion, we must remain aware that it is not enough to simply measure survival from time of diagnosis; we need some other way to measure a test's effects on life expectancy.

We might initially look for the answer in national breast cancer mortality statistics: Are there fewer deaths from breast cancer since the introduction of mammography? Yet such statistics may not answer our questions about the benefits of mammography, for a variety of reasons. Perhaps other factors are affecting the incidence, detection, or treatment of disease at the same time that the change in screening practices is taking place. Furthermore, national data on mortality do not tell us who is being screened and whether the screened women are living longer.

What would be an appropriate way to measure the benefits of mammography accurately? Presumably, the earlier diagnosis made possible by screening should lead to earlier treatment and either a cure or prolonged

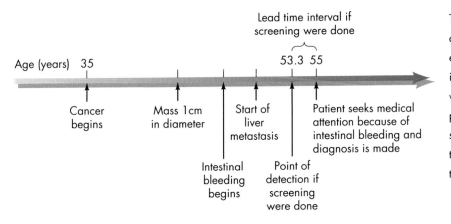

Age (years) 35

Cancer begins

Mass 1cm in diameter

Start of liver metastasis

Intestinal bleeding begins

Point of detection if screening were done

Lead time interval if screening were done

53.3 55

Patient seeks medical attention because of intestinal bleeding and diagnosis is made

This diagram of the events leading to the detection of colon cancer illustrates that earlier screening may lead to an increase in the time between detection and death, whether or not earlier treatment succeeds in postponing the date of death. A study assessing the impact of screening on survival time has to take into account the extra lead time introduced by earlier detection.

life. The best way to measure the effect of a screening program on decreased mortality from breast cancer is to conduct a randomized clinical trial, assigning some people to the new screening program and others to the standard pattern of care. The HIP study of mammography has set the standard for this type of evaluation. In the 1960s, 62,000 women members of HIP, a comprehensive, prepaid medical insurance plan, were identified for study. Women were allocated to treatment and control groups based on their insurance identification numbers, which were unrelated to any personal characteristics. Women in the study group received an initial mammographic screening and three annual follow-up mammograms. Women in the control group followed the plan's established pattern of care, which included general physical examinations. In either group, physicians referred women for biopsy if indicated and to treatment if necessary.

After the first five years, 304 cases of breast cancer were diagnosed in the study group, compared to 298 cases in the control group. The cases in the study group appeared to be less severe; 32 percent showed histologic evidence of the cancer spreading to the axillary lymph nodes, compared to 42 percent in the control group. After ten years there was a cumulative total of 95 deaths from breast cancer in the study group, as against 133 deaths in the control group. It appeared that screening had resulted in earlier treatment of breast cancer and had saved 38 lives.

The HIP study found that the control group (those with standard clinical exams) had more breast cancer deaths within a ten-year period than did the study group (those with regular mammograms). Moreover, deaths from breast cancer in the control group occurred sooner after the start of the study than did deaths in the study group.

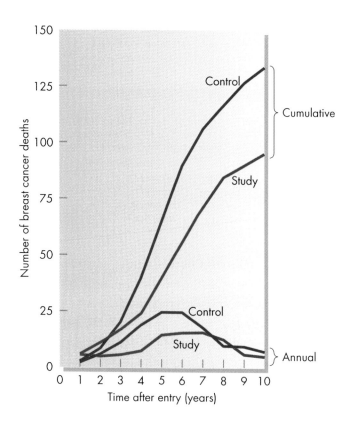

Regular mammography screenings were demonstrated to confer benefits on women who entered the study at age 50 and over, but did not appear to confer benefits on women aged 40 to 49 at entry. After five years there were 19 and 20 cumulative deaths to women aged 40 to 49 in the study and control groups, respectively (see the table on the facing page). After ten years, when the entire group was over 50, some differences in mortality begin to appear: there were 39 breast cancer deaths in the study group, and 51 breast cancer deaths in the control group.

Deciding How to Use a Screening Test

THE United States Preventive Services Task Force has recommended the following with regard to mammography and clinical examinations: "All women over age 40 should receive an annual clinical breast examination.

Cumulative Numbers of Breast Cancer Deaths among Cases of Breast Cancer in the HIP Study

Age at entry (years)	Time after entry					
	5 years		10 years		18 years	
	Study	Control	Study	Control	Study	Control
40–49	19	20	39	51	49	65
50–59	15	33	42	61	57	74
60–64	5	10	14	21	20	24
Total	39	63	95	133	126	163

Mammography every one to two years is recommended for all women beginning at age 50 and concluding at approximately age 75 unless pathology had been detected. It may be prudent to begin mammography at an earlier age for women at high risk for breast cancer." In their accompanying discussion the task force pointed out that the benefits for women aged 40 to 49 have not been demonstrated. The task force estimated the annual cost of mammography for women aged 40 and over to be $2 billion (in 1984), not counting the cost of biopsies for women with false positive mammograms. They assessed the variation in radiation levels associated with mammograms, as well as variation in quality of mammography. In addition, they considered the burden of this disease—the large number of women affected by and dying of breast cancer.

The questions taken up, which can be summarized as follows, provide an excellent scheme for evaluating any medical screening procedure or program. What is the purpose of the particular screening procedure? What are its sensitivity and its specificity? How much does the test cost? How serious is the disease for which the test screens? What are the consequences of being mislabeled as positive? Is the screening test painful or dangerous? Is treatment for the condition available?

The purpose of mammography, reduction of mortality, appears to be accomplished in women over 50, but not in younger women. The test sensitivity is adequate in women over 50, and specificity is good. However, mammography may be more costly than is desired for a population-wide screening procedure, and it incurs costs for women with false positives, both in worry and in the medical expense of biopsy. The discomfort occasioned by mammography is brief; the risk that the radiation exposure the test involves will itself cause cancer is low, and improved technology is minimizing it. Breast cancer is a serious disease, and treatment is available for women with insurance, living near moderate-to-large medical facilities.

Although epidemiology can contribute information and interpret data, each party involved (physician, patient, insurer, etc.) will give different weights to each fact, despite going through similar processes in reviewing the information, and may wind up with somewhat differing conclusions. The American Cancer Society and the National Cancer Institute recommended baseline mammography from ages 35 to 40, annual or biennial mammograms from ages 40 to 49, and annual mammograms beginning at age 50. Groups such as the American Medical Association, the American College of Obstetricians and Gynecologists, and the American College of Radiology supported these recommendations, but other medical associations (the Canadian Task Force, the American College of Physicians) recommended that mammography begin at age 50. Even after we develop policy recommendations, moreover, we need to separate general issues from individual clinical needs. In this vein, the U.S. Preventive Services Task Force noted that "for the special category of women at high risk because of family history . . . it may be prudent to begin . . . mammography at an earlier age."

Genetic Screening

THANKS to exciting developments in molecular biology, it has now become possible to screen for disease-causing genetic mutations, perhaps years or even decades before the first symptoms of disease appear. Although testing for genetic diseases began in the 1960s with the screening of newborns for phenylketonuria (PKU, a metabolic disorder that causes mental retardation if not prevented by a change in diet), such tests identi-

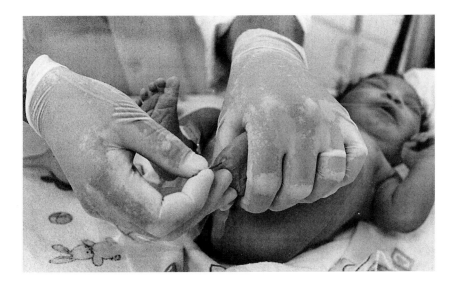

A simple heel prick produces a drop of blood for the routine screening of newborns—mandatory in many states—for the metabolic disorder phenylketonuria (PKU). Mental retardation is the likely result of PKU if the disorder is not detected immediately and treated.

fied disease-caused abnormalities: proteins that reflected the metabolic errors caused by the gene. Present-day technology allows us to look at the genome itself to note the presence or absence of a given gene, and even to describe the particular type of mutation found. As the mapping of the human genome continues at an intense pace, the genes for various diseases will be discovered with increasing frequency (some recent examples are the genes for Huntington's disease, breast cancer, and cystic fibrosis). With the discovery of each new gene, the question immediately arises how to use a test for the gene in clinical practice and community screening.

Although the goal of screening has traditionally been to prevent disease, or at least reduce its impact, treatment is not always available for the conditions uncovered by genetic screening. If a fetus is discovered to have a disease-causing genetic mutation, its parents may decide to terminate the pregnancy. People who discover that they carry a gene for an untreatable illness can acquire information that can help them plan their lives, their finances, their reproductive choices, and other behaviors. Providing information has itself become the stated goal of genetic screening.

Genetic screening tests, like other screening tests, have imperfect sensitivity, specificity, and predictive value. Occasionally their results

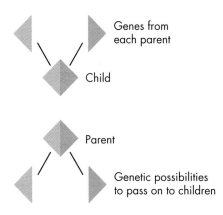

Genes from
each parent

Child

Parent

Genetic possibilities
to pass on to children

Top: We each have two copies of every gene, one from our father and one from our mother, although we may inherit different variants of the gene from each parent (for example, one copy could carry cystic fibrosis and the other not). Bottom: We pass on only one of our two copies of a gene to each child, so a parent carrying one copy of the cystic fibrosis variant (the other copy of that gene is healthy) has a 50 percent chance of donating the disease variant to his or her child.

may be inaccurate because of limitations in laboratory techniques, variations in the mutations for a given gene, and the presence of other factors that influence the gene's activity and the eventual development of disease. Overall, though, the accuracy and predictive value of genetic screening tests are much higher than those attained by previous medical screening tests. Variations in the mutations for a given gene can lower sensitivity and complicate the screening process. Although a single faulty gene is often enough to cause an inherited illness, the flaw in that gene can be the result of any one of many possible mutations. The recent history of the debate over screening for cystic fibrosis illustrates how the existence of different mutations can introduce a complication that must then be addressed by epidemiologic studies.

Cystic fibrosis is a disease that manifests itself in frequent coughing, lung infections, and difficulty breathing. Although often diagnosed in the first year of life, people with the disease may live into their thirties. An individual develops cystic fibrosis when he or she inherits two copies of the gene for the disease, one from the mother and one from the father. People with one gene for the disease are carriers, but do not themselves develop the illness. If two carriers conceive a child together, they each have a 50 percent chance of passing on the gene, and the combined probability that they will both pass on the gene for cystic fibrosis (and that their child will have the illness) is 25 percent.

When the gene for cystic fibrosis was cloned in 1989, the medical community seemed poised to implement widespread screening for the gene, but instituting a screening program turned out to be far more complicated than expected. Lap-Chu Tsui at the University of Michigan had found a gene mutation that seemed to cause most cases of cystic fibrosis. Tsui expected that the mutations causing the remaining cases could be found within one year, and to that end he coordinated a collaborative effort among nearly 70 laboratories around the world. The laboratories immediately turned up 20 rare mutations, but these mutations together accounted for only a small percentage of the remaining cases. Indeed, most of the mutations were found only among the members of single families. By trying out the test for the first gene mutation on parents of people with cystic fibrosis, the scientists were able to establish that Tsui's mutation

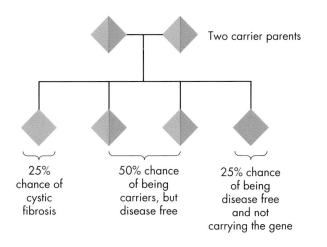

Two carrier parents

25% chance of cystic fibrosis

50% chance of being carriers, but disease free

25% chance of being disease free and not carrying the gene

The pattern of inheritance for cystic fibrosis. Two carrier parents have a 25 percent chance of conceiving a child who will have cystic fibrosis.

predicted only 75 percent of the carriers of cystic fibrosis—that is, the sensitivity of the test was 75 percent, significantly lower than the desired value of 95 percent.

At the present time, more than sixty mutations have been discovered, each accounting for a small percentage of the people with cystic fibrosis and each requiring a separate genetic screening test. In 1990, the National Institute of Health Workshop on Population Screening for the Cystic Fibrosis Gene recommended against screening the population at large until the hoped-for 95 percent sensitivity was in reach. In light of this unexpected development, the NIH workshop urged that pilot studies be developed to study how best to implement screening for cystic fibrosis.

The epidemiologists carrying out the studies had to address the questions, how could the population to be tested be narrowed to a manageable size? Should programs target couples planning to have children, or instead should they target relatives of people with cystic fibrosis? Should people be screened even if they are not planning on having children? Epidemiologists also wanted find out how people would accept an imperfect genetic test.

Two studies in Great Britain evaluated different strategies for offering screening to people who might have the gene for cystic fibrosis. M. Super

Dr. Tsui, the scientist who discovered the mutation that accounts for 75 percent of the cases of cystic fibrosis, shown in his laboratory at the Hospital for Sick Children, Toronto, examining a DNA analysis.

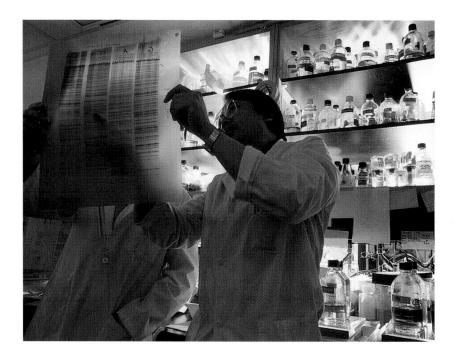

and colleagues in Manchester, England, evaluated a program screening the relatives and partners of 607 people affected with cystic fibrosis. Of 1,563 people tested, 15 couples were found to be at risk of having a child with the disease (that is, both members of the couple had the gene for cystic fibrosis). The women in nine of these couples were pregnant; eight then had prenatal tests, and of the eight, four were found to be carrying an affected fetus. Three of the four women terminated their pregnancies. In June 1994, the authors concluded that screening relatives was an effective way of identifying carrier couples.

During that same month, Jean Livingstone and her colleagues presented the results of a pilot program that targeted couples rather than relatives. They offered screening to all couples visiting two prenatal clinics in Edinburgh, Scotland, regardless of whether the couples had relatives with cystic fibrosis. They approached 8,536 couples, 714 of whom were ineligible because prenatal care began late in pregnancy and 1,900 of whom declined. Among the 5,922 couples screened, four were identified as at risk (each partner carried the gene for cystic fibrosis). All four chose to have their fetuses tested; two women were carrying fetuses with two copies of the gene for cystic fibrosis, and both pregnancies were terminated. The investigators had to screen 5,922 couples (or 11,844 people) to find four couples at risk of having an affected child, compared to the 1,563 people screened by Super and colleagues to find fifteen affected couples.

In both pilot programs, couples were free to decline screening for themselves or their fetuses, in accord with the stated goal of genetic screening to provide people with information that they can then use in conformance with their own values and beliefs. A couple who know they are carriers can prepare for the possibility of an infant with cystic fibrosis, or the couple can consider options such as adoption, artificial insemination, and abortion. Both pilot programs demonstrated that people take different approaches when confronted with their carrier status or the news that their child will be born with a life-threatening disease.

Epidemiologists will continue to evaluate the impact of genetic screening programs, but society as a whole will decide on the ultimate uses of genetic screening. Although the scientific and medical communities have urged the delay of population-wide screening for cystic fibrosis until pilot studies were completed, an estimated 9,310 tests were performed in the United States in 1991 and an estimated 63,000 in 1992. This last number still represents only about 0.6 percent of the 10 million people seen annually for prenatal care. As cystic fibrosis screening becomes more common, law courts may begin to find physicians liable if they do not offer screening to couples that later give birth to a child with the disease. The use of the test may thus develop its own momentum, and become part of standard care. In this fast-paced world, epidemiologic data may be temporarily pushed aside, but in the long run epidemiologic studies will continue to play a role in providing society with information necessary for planning genetic screening programs.

New Procedures — New Demands

EPIDEMIOLOGISTS can provide information about a test's sensitivity, specificity, and predictive value; about patients who would benefit from being screened, and about the health and financial consequences of screening. But the final use to which a screening test is put depends not just on the scientific data, but on economic pressures and social values. Advocacy groups like the American Heart Association and the American Cancer Society generally support screening for "their" diseases, and create a demand for screening tests by spreading information. Patients, for their part, are often glad of the opportunity to put their minds at rest regarding their personal risk of a specific condition. When pharmaceutical companies and health care providers also advertise the availability of screening procedures, the demand for a screening test may become irresistible before epidemiologists have had the chance to offer a thorough analysis of the test's benefits.

How a combination of economic pressures and advocacy can force a particular diagnostic procedure into general practice before a study can even be made is illustrated by the history of the blood test for prostatic specific antigen (PSA). The simple test, incorporated into a battery of routine tests, costs from $50 to $80 and may allow earlier detection of prostate cancer than can be obtained by physical examination. At the test's introduction in 1989, market forces quickly began to enter the decision whether to screen men on a broad basis. Drug companies, medical supply houses, the American Cancer Society, and other groups have publicized the issue of prostate cancer screening to such a degree that PSA screening has almost established itself as routine in the care of men over 50. Yet the value of the test remains uncertain, and it is likely to be difficult to study the question in a randomized clinical trial in this country, since it may prove impossible to find a sufficiently large population of men who consent to be allocated to study groups not receiving PSA screening.

Economic forces may also operate to discourage testing. The debate over screening becomes especially heated when health care costs are considered. Screening tests are done on large numbers of people and, when multiplied many times over, involve huge sums of money. Furthermore, they can generate increased use of specialized equipment (like the x-ray machines used in mammography) and, often, the need to order additional tests to confirm or refute the initial reading in the group that tested positive. Thus, insurers may not wish to pay for the costs of screening, especially if they fail to see a proportionate decrease in costs paid for medical care for the particular disease in question. Lack of insurance coverage for a screening test may then affect a person's decision to have the test done.

Many people believe that the expenditure of personnel, equipment, money, and patient time on screening procedures will be outweighed by savings in resources allocated to treatment of advanced disease, although this may not always be true. The prophylactic options generated by some screening tests can be quite expensive, as in the example of women with a gene for breast cancer who elect to undergo radical mastectomies. The issues of information, cost, and disease prevention are all ingredients in the debate over the use of screening tests, their uses, and who should pay for them. Further intensifying the debate are concerns over the confidentiality of information and the legal concepts of standard care. The outcome of such debates reflects cultural values and social pressures and will continue to influence screening programs just as surely as will the epidemiological data itself.

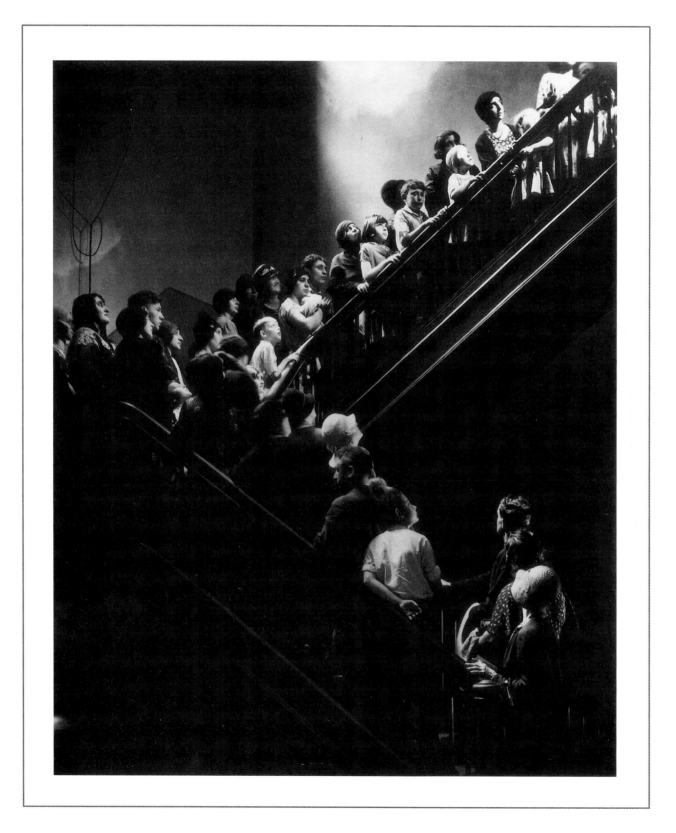

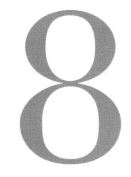

Health Care Services:
What Works?

"ON THE Clinic Stairs," photographed by Edward
Steichen. The evaluation of public health programs,
and the distinguishing of effective activities from
useless ones, is one of epidemiology's critically
important tasks.

Epidemiology makes another of its contributions to medical research by organizing the collection of health information and formulating questions, based on statistical analysis of this data, that will help to explore and improve the workings of the health care system. Florence Nightingale, whose work was described in Chapter 2, was an effective model for the epidemiologist's systematic scrutiny of the organized delivery of health care—in her case, within British Army hospitals and at the front. Today the issues are both more numerous and more complex. Many public, private, and nonprofit organizations and agencies offer medical treatment and information. Some medical decisions may be decisively influenced by religious or political beliefs, such as those concerning abortion or the "right to die." Others may depend on issues of finance: Will an insurance policy, a drug company, or a government program pay for a given treatment (especially if the therapy is rare, costly, or experimental)? Legal guidelines may come into play.

Epidemiology, by the nature of its detachment from these issues and reliance on the scientific method, can keep medical objectives and outcomes in focus. It can evaluate courses of treatment (whether they rely on drugs or on surgery), guidelines for clinical practice, and organized delivery of preventive and therapeutic information and active interventions. It can investigate how people feel about their health and their health care services. Finally, having identified medical goals and appropriate practice, it can contribute vital information to the ongoing social process of weighing what the public's health requires against the resources available to meet those needs.

Program Evaluation: The Case of Parkinsonism

IT is vitally important to medicine to learn what works—to separate those drugs, surgical procedures, and other treatments that are most efficacious from those that lack benefit. The risks and costs incurred by useless treatments are to be avoided in favor of the worthwhile and practical. This seemingly simple principle is easier to state than to implement. One

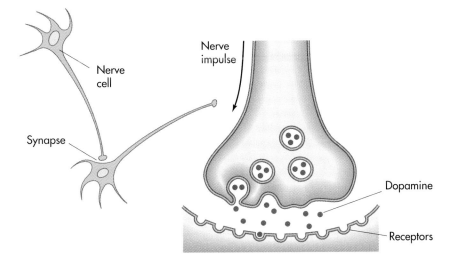

An electrical signal, or nerve impulse, travels through an activated nerve cell until it reaches the "synapse" between two cells. The arrival of the signal stimulates the release of a chemical substance called a neurotransmitter into the synapse; the neurotransmitter in turn stimulates a nerve impulse in the neighboring nerve cell. In Parkinson's disease, the loss of nerve cells in the substantia nigra that produce the neurotransmitter dopamine means that some nerve signals are not transmitted. This loss causes the characteristic symptoms of rigid movement, slowness of movement, and "pill-rolling" tremor of the hands. Eventually, difficulty with swallowing and walking take their toll on the victims of this rather common neurological disorder of unknown cause.

modern example dramatically illustrates this difficulty: Does the drug selegiline (Eldepryl) prevent the progression of Parkinson's disease?

Parkinson's disease is a debilitating movement disorder whose onset is insidious but tends to begin in middle age. It grows worse over the years, as tremors and muscular rigidity lead to physical incapacity and, often, dementia. Parkinsonism is the result of depleted neurotransmitters in the midbrain; these are the chemical substances that transmit signals from nerve cell to nerve cell. Drugs such as L-dopa (levodopa) can provide a partial replacement that abates some symptoms. But the causes of this depletion are varied and sometimes mysterious; they include carbon monoxide poisoning, head injury, cerebral arteriosclerosis, and encephalitis.

The drug selegiline has been advocated to slow the progress of this disease. Selegiline was developed after a mini-epidemic of Parkinson's disease was noted in California in the mid-1970s, related to ingestion of an illicit "designer" drug, MPTP. This synthetic street drug destroys neurons located in the substantia nigra region of the midbrain, causing the rapid onset of severe, chemically induced Parkinson's disease. This environmentally caused Parkinsonism paradoxically contributed a strong tool to researchers studying this illness since the disease could now be induced in experimental animals by administering MPTP. Once the animal model was created, drugs could be tested to see if they could block the onset of disease after the animals were given MPTP. One of these drugs, selegiline, seemed to work in the experimental animals. But does it work in human Parkinson's disease patients?

Questions about selegiline's efficacy in humans are particularly important because the drug has some nasty side effects and is expensive. If it does not do the job, then both risk and cost are incurred for no benefit; if it does do the job, it should be promoted and prescribed for virtually all early cases of Parkinson's disease. As we write, this question is still unanswered in a convincing way; early Parkinson's disease patients must make a decision whether or not to use this drug with very incomplete evidence to guide them and their physicians.

The ideal research design to address this question is a randomized controlled clinical trial. Eligible subjects (patients with early Parkinson's disease) would be randomly assigned to one of two groups, one receiving selegiline and one receiving a placebo. The trial would ideally be double-blinded—neither the patients nor the assessing physicians would know whether any given patient was taking the active or inert drug. Double-blinding reduces opportunities for the operation of bias in the assessment of results. The randomization procedure, moreover, further reduces the chance of a biased assignment of any patient to one of the two groups, thus assuring comparability between the groups: any difference that

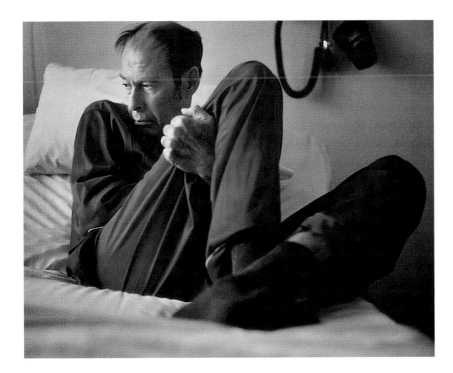

This man is disabled by Parkinson's disease. The drug L-dopa is the only really effective reliever of symptoms, but because large, controlled clinical trials have never been carried out it is unclear whether the drug should be first administered early in the disease or only after significant disability develops.

emerges can be reliably attributed to the drug rather than to the prior condition of the patient.

Such a trial was carried out in Europe in 1993. Benefit was measured by calculating the length of time patients were well enough to avoid taking L-dopa, currently the most effective drug for treating Parkinson's disease. The study's results unfortunately were equivocal, showing very modest benefit: about a six-month delay before having to begin taking L-dopa was achieved by the groups on selegiline as contrasted to the group on placebo. It is not clear, however, if this delay was due to selegiline's ability to retard progression of the disease or to its mild anti-Parkinsonian pharmacologic action—that is, selegiline may have treated the very mildest Parkinson's disease symptoms, rather than retarding or preventing their onset. With this question still moot, and with the benefit apparently so slight, neurologists are divided as to what to advise early Parkinson's disease patients.

Program Evaluation: Examples in Surgical Treatment

SURGERY often involves even greater risks than do drugs, so it is especially important to test not only proposed new surgical procedures but also older, established surgical treatment to ensure its efficacy and weigh this against the risks of the surgery itself. The importance of using the randomized controlled trial to accomplish this objective was vividly illustrated in a classic paper written by Thomas Chalmers and his colleagues almost forty years ago. It evaluated the evidence put forth by surgeons to persuade their colleagues to adopt procedures they had pioneered for the treatment of portal hypertension, a life-threatening consequence of alcoholic cirrhosis of the liver.

Portal hypertension occurs when veins in the liver become clogged by the scarring of the liver that results from damage by alcohol. The blood flow becomes backed up, and the blood pressure raised, in the portal vein and its tributaries feeding into the liver from the intestines. A result is the accumulation of fluid in the abdominal cavity (a condition called ascites) and, eventually, coma. A series of operations called "shunts" were developed by surgeons to relieve this pressure in the portal venous system. One popular shunt attached the portal vein to the inferior vena cava, the main vein draining the abdominal cavity and organs.

These Draconian surgical procedures were reported by their inventors and advocates to provide marked relief to patients who underwent them. Most of these enthusiastic reports, however, took the form of uncontrolled case series. Some were reports of a series of patients who had the shunts, compared to a set of controls, but where no randomization was used in assigning patients to one group or the other. And only a few of the reports were of randomized controlled trials.

The Chalmers study summarized these reports and analyzed the results according to type of research design. It emerged from this analysis that the case series carried out without controls allowed the most enthusiastic interpretation of results and were uniformly favorable to the new surgical procedures. When a control group was incorporated into the design, the interpretation become more guarded and cautious. And when a randomized controlled study design was employed, the procedures were

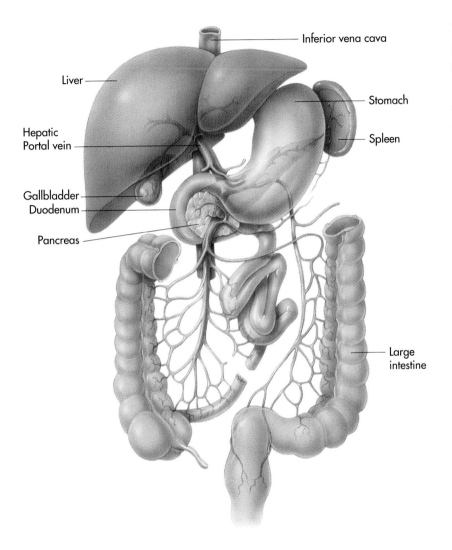

Inferior vena cava

Liver

Hepatic
Portal vein

Gallbladder
Duodenum

Pancreas

Stomach

Spleen

Large
intestine

The portal vein and its tributaries carry the products of digestion from the intestines to the liver, where those products are further metabolized. Cirrhosis of the liver, with its destruction of tissue and scarring, eventually leads to blocked circulation of the liver and portal hypertension. The obstructed blood flow may back up in the portal system of veins, resulting in ascites or even, in some cases, rupture and massive hemorrhage.

generally reported to be of no benefit. This analysis led to the facetious promulgation of the law that states that when a surgical procedure is of no benefit whatever, a case series without a control group must be used to produce the illusion of benefit.

Another famous trial of a surgical intervention put its efficacy to the crucial test and led to the demise of the procedure. In the early 1960s a gastric freezing technique was developed for the treatment of bleeding

This ulcer in the stomach lining of a rat has the classic punched-out appearance and smooth base typical of these breaks in tissue. If the ulcer extends deep enough to erode a blood vessel, the ulcer will bleed.

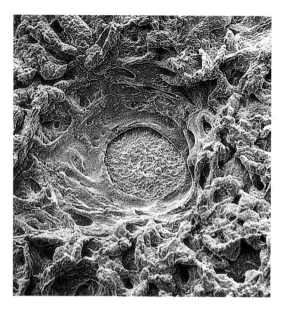

gastric or duodenal ulcers: A famous surgeon, experimenting with this technique using sheep, had seemed to show that if a tube attached to a deflated balloon was passed into the stomach and the balloon was later inflated and filled with a freezing solution, this reliably stopped the bleeding from the ulcer.

A case series of over 80 patients was reported by this surgeon. He claimed success even though there was no control group for comparison. This article received a great deal of attention, and special gastric freezing machines were manufactured and sold. One of the present authors (Paul Stolley), as an intern at a university hospital, actually administered gastric freezing to a patient with bleeding ulcers.

The National Institutes of Health were concerned that this new and relatively untested treatment was becoming so widely adopted before adequate proof of efficacy had been presented. They therefore organized, in 1963, a randomized controlled clinical trial using a sham procedure group as a control. Those patients randomized to receive the sham procedure swallowed a balloon just as did the gastric freeze group; however, the solution placed in the balloon never reached a freezing temperature—but neither patient nor assessing physician could tell who had received the true freeze and who had received the sham.

Results were disappointing but not unexpected: the group receiving the freeze did no better than the group receiving the sham procedure. Indeed, over many months the true freeze group did worse, having more recurrences than the sham group. It is thought that the freezing solution may have damaged the stomach tissues, making a recurrence of ulcers more likely.

Some Surprising Results from Public Health Campaigns

THE same issue of evaluation relevant to drugs and surgery applies as well to large public health programs. Does addition of fluoride to the public water supply reduce the amount of tooth decay? Does screening for breast cancer by use of mammography reduce breast cancer mortality (or does it merely pick up the tumors at an earlier stage without cutting down on the actual death rate)? Does the mass campaign to teach children and adults to swim reduce the number of deaths from drowning? Do programs to educate drivers result in more seat belt use? And do seat belts, when used, lower the rate of fatalities due to automobile accidents?

When rigorous scientific methods of evaluation are applied to established health programs, they sometimes demonstrate their clear efficacy, as is the case with fluoridation of the water supply or the properly buckled seat belt. But there may be unpleasant and unexpected surprises. The example of the antidrowning campaign is instructive. For many years the American Red Cross stressed swimming instruction as a means of preventing drownings; but in spite of these efforts, the rate of drowning increased. An epidemiological study was carried out in the state of Maryland, examining all drownings that occurred during the summer of 1975. It was found that most persons who drowned at the beach *did* know how to swim; in fact, nonswimmers seldom ventured into the water above their knees.

What tended to distinguish persons who drowned from those who did not (using the case-control design described in Chapter 3) was not their ability to swim but rather their consumption of alcohol before going in the water. Alcohol ingestion was the risk factor of greatest import for drowning. The Red Cross, by teaching more people to swim, had in a sense put more people at risk of drowning. The important educational message should have been: never drink and swim, just as you should not drink and drive. Both swimming and driving require complex motor coordination skills that are seriously compromised by drinking alcohol.

Similarly, a campaign to persuade the residents of a large Midwestern city to use seat belts while driving was launched using television, newspaper, radio, and billboard messages. The campaign saturated the media for three months, but a survey of drivers before, during, and after the campaign showed little change in seat belt use (about 20 percent of drivers used them at all three periods measured). Then the state in which this city is located passed a law requiring seat belt use and imposed a fine on anyone stopped by the police for some reason and found not wearing them. Usage jumped to about 80 percent and stayed there. If these two approaches to encouraging seat belt use had not been rigorously evaluated, we might still be attempting to increase this lifesaving practice with the ineffective educational approach instead of the much more successful legislative approach. While health education intuitively seems so reasonable and is less offensive to most people than legal action, it is often less effective. Health services research, which permits public health scientists to discover what works best, is crucial to informed policy formulation.

Clinical Decision Making under Epidemiology's Lens

EPIDEMIOLOGISTS are increasingly devoting their attention to the description and analysis of problems of clinical medicine. Why, for example, is the hysterectomy rate so high in the United States? It is about six times the Swedish rate, three times the rate in the United Kingdom, and double the Canadian rate. Is this because of the presence in the United States of more cases of the clinical conditions for which hysterectomy must be performed, or is the high rate due rather to this country's lax indications for the procedure and different surgical practice styles? What, moreover, is the benefit of this high rate of surgery?

A recent study suggests that about 15 percent of hysterectomies performed in the United States are clearly not medically justified, while another 25 percent are performed for unclear or vague medical indications. Hysterectomies in Maryland have been thoroughly studied over a ten-year period by Kristin Kjerullf and her colleagues, revealing interesting differences according to patients' race. The median age for hysterectomy in Maryland is more than five years younger for African American women (36 years) than for their Caucasian counterparts (41 years), and among African Americans, more than two-thirds of these surgeries are performed for uterine fibroids, whereas in Caucasian Maryland women less than 40 percent of hysterectomies are performed for fibroids. Patterns of surgery, both national and international, can be investigated using epidemiologic methods to help understand why they differ so greatly and whether improved criteria can be developed to guide surgeons and women in making decisions.

Tonsillectomy used to be the most common surgical procedure performed in the United States. During the 1940s the majority of children in some communities underwent this operation, which was advocated to prevent pharyngitis (sore throats) and upper respiratory infections. Randomized controlled clinical trials, finally carried out in the mid-1970s to evaluate this common surgical operation, were disappointing. These results, combined with the advent of antibiotics to treat pharyngitis and eradicate streptococcus bacteria, led to a gradual decline in the frequency with which this procedure was performed; this in turn resulted in the closure of some hospitals for children and a decrease in the number of hospital bed-days that children utilized.

At the height of its popularity, however, tonsillectomy was thought (without adequate evidence) to be so valuable that a group of social activists were concerned that poor children were being deprived of this operation. To demonstrate the problem they arranged to have a large number of children from an impoverished district of New York City examined at school by pediatric ear, nose, and throat specialists to determine whether the procedure was indicated. The figure on the following page shows the results of the examinations of these children by three such groups of doctors.

A New York City program of the mid-1940s sent 389 children to be evaluated for tonsillectomy by up to three physicians. All children ruled not in need of a tonsillectomy by the first physician were reexamined by a second physician; those still considered not in need of a tonsillectomy were screened by yet a third physician. All three doctors referred about the same percentage of children for tonsillectomy, suggesting that they based their recommendations on expectations rather than on objective, validated criteria.

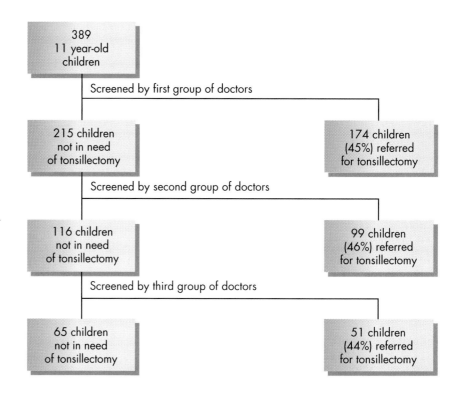

389
11 year-old children

Screened by first group of doctors

215 children not in need of tonsillectomy

174 children (45%) referred for tonsillectomy

Screened by second group of doctors

116 children not in need of tonsillectomy

99 children (46%) referred for tonsillectomy

Screened by third group of doctors

65 children not in need of tonsillectomy

51 children (44%) referred for tonsillectomy

It is clear from this figure that criteria for this surgery were so loose that almost any child, if examined by enough surgeons, would have a tonsillectomy recommended. Indeed, the mere "presence of tonsils" might be sufficient grounds to recommend the operation. Studies have shown that the appearance of a child's tonsils and history of past infection were ordinarily the basis for the decision to operate. These were factors so vaguely described and their definitions so unclear that any two surgeons might have very different "decision rules" about the operation and when to perform it. And none of the decision rules or algorithms was based on good information, as few reliable comparative studies had ever been carried out. In retrospect, it seems remarkable that an operation could become so widespread based on so little supporting empirical data. The "fee-for-service" method of payment then prevalent and insurance companies' failure to demand better evidence for the procedure probably contributed to its popularity. One of the authors of this volume (Paul Stolley) had two tonsillectomies in childhood (the first one was apparently incomplete) and has vivid memories of the anesthesia and pain he underwent at the age of five.

The Uncertainty of Clinical Decision Making: The Case of Prostate Cancer

LOOKING at single examples of an overused surgical procedure or at an inadequately evaluated drug cannot give us a true conception of the complexity of the decisions encountered by the physician and patient facing a serious illness. There can be, in fact, a whole series of decisions to be made—concerning how to screen, diagnose, and treat the ailment. Moreover, the information available about any one procedure in the series (how truly effective it is) will influence earlier or later decisions. As an example, the diagnosis and treatment of prostate cancer present several knotty problems that have only begun to be solved through the efforts of epidemiologists.

In the past few years it has become routine to test the blood of middle-aged men for an elevated level of prostatic specific antigen (PSA), one of the many substances secreted by the prostate gland. This test is now advocated by many urologists and oncologists as a way to detect prostate cancer in its earliest stage so that the tumor can be treated, and perhaps cured, with surgery, radiation, or drugs. The costs of this screening effort can be very great in time, money, and even, occasionally, injury to the patient (if a false positive leads to an unnecessary procedure). But if it is effective, it could cut the toll of human suffering for a cancer that is now the third leading cause of cancer death in American men, after lung cancer and colon cancer.

A man eventually diagnosed with prostate cancer will go through an entire sequence of procedures:

1. The PSA test is performed; if the PSA level is high, the test is repeated.
2. If the level is still high on the repeat test, a physician performs a rectal digital exam to palpate part of the prostate in search of tumors and an ultrasound exam to image the prostate gland.

3. If the ultrasound or rectal digital exam reveals a suspicious area that could be a tumor, a biopsy is performed to obtain a sample of gland tissue.
4. The tissue is examined under a microscope by a pathologist: it may or may not reveal cancer.
5. If the tissue is "read" as cancer, a treatment must be decided upon: surgery, radiation, drugs, or "watchful waiting."

The problem with this sequence of events is that there is great uncertainty about almost every step. The PSA test, being relatively new and not adequately studied, has not had its accuracy properly characterized. Its sensitivity and specificity are not yet well described—that is, the proportion of all tests that are routinely false positives and the proportion that are routinely false negatives is still unclear.

The diagnostic steps following a positive test are also problematic. The rectal digital exam is a crude technique that misses tumors not in a location where the examiner's finger can feel them. The sonogram produced by the ultrasound exam is more accurate and the risk attached to it is insignificant, but again its sensitivity and specificity have not been adequately characterized. Are all suspicious images that will lead to a biopsy truly called positive? And if not, what proportion of seemingly positive tests are actually false?

If the sonogram reveals a possible tumor, then the next step is a prostate biopsy. A needle is guided into the suspicious area and a pinch of tissue (or several) is obtained for examination under a microscope. This procedure is not merely often uncomfortable, but can result in bleeding or infection. Moreover, although a biopsy can determine the presence of a cancer, it does not resolve all questions. It appears that prostate cancer can stay indolent for a long time in some persons, for reasons that are not known; but in others the tumors can be aggressive and quickly metastasize (spreading usually to bone), causing great discomfort, bone fractures, and eventually death. The terrible problem faced by pathologists is that they cannot tell whether a tumor will be aggressive or indolent with any great degree of predictive validity just by looking at tissue under the microscope. Therefore, the tissue's appearance may not help guide

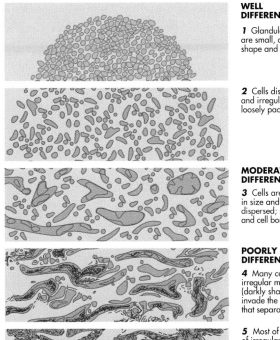

WELL DIFFERENTIATED

1 Glandular (secretory) cells are small, of fairly uniform shape and tightly packed.

2 Cells display more varied and irregular shapes and are loosely packed.

MODERATELY DIFFERENTIATED

3 Cells are even more irregular in size and shape and are more dispersed; some cells are fused, and cell borders are less distinct.

POORLY DIFFERENTIATED

4 Many cells are fused into irregular masses; some cells (darkly shaded) have begun to invade the connective tissue that separates cells.

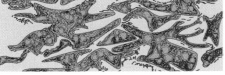

5 Most of the tumor consists of irregular masses that have invaded the connective tissue.

Pathologists believe they can find clues to the aggressiveness of prostate tumors in the size, shape, and appearance of cancerous cells. Those cells that are well differentiated like normal tissue are considered less aggressive, yet some cancers that appear benign turn out to be metastatic.

treatment. There is little way to tell which is best, watchful waiting or aggressive surgery.

Finally, the cure rates of the various treatments are not known because few comparative controlled clinical trials have been carried out. Lest we think the problem of surgery carried out without clear evidence of its benefits and risks is a purely historical phenomenon, consider the current controversy about the value of radical prostatectomy (removal of the gland surgically) for carcinoma of the prostate. It is still not known whether or not this surgical procedure is a worthwhile operation. Does it improve survivorship, lower mortality, or improve the quality of life of those men with prostate cancer who undergo it? How does it compare to alternative medical therapies such as hormone treatment, radiation, or both? Since the operation has significant morbidity attached to it and can also result in incontinence and impotence, these are important considerations for doctor and patient. Randomized controlled trials of this surgical procedure are now underway, although results are not available as of the time this volume goes to press.

Consider the dilemma of the patient who is told that his PSA test is "borderline high" and in fact higher than his test of the previous year. He must then decide if he will pursue the search for a possible prostate tumor. If he chooses to have the sonogram, it may lead to a biopsy; the biopsy may result in a diagnosis of prostate cancer, and he may then be faced with choosing a therapy without the evidence needed to guide his choice. If he chooses watchful waiting, the tumor may stay in the prostate gland, remaining small and not metastasizing (as is often the case). But there is always the danger that the tumor will escape the confines of the gland and move to bone. Even if the patient chooses the most radical treatment—a prostatectomy—he is choosing a procedure for which the cure rate is unknown but the side effects in the form of impotence and incontinence can be considerable.

Very recently, however, a study reported encouraging results about the sensitivity and specificity of the PSA test. The study was what is called a "nested" case-control study within a long-term randomized controlled trial of men designed to test the efficacy of aspirin in the prevention of myocardial infarction. As part of the aspirin study, blood samples from all the men were kept frozen and preserved for future use, and the development of new cancers was noted. Eventually the investigators obtained blood samples for 366 men who had developed prostate cancer. For each case, they selected three controls who had not reported a diagnosis of prostate cancer and whose age matched that of the case to within one year. The PSA test was applied to blood samples that had been obtained at the beginning of the study for both the cases and controls. Meanwhile, one of the investigators made a "blind" review of the medical records of the prostate cancer cases and categorized the cases by stage (degree of spread) and microscopic appearance as "aggressive" or "nonaggressive." Comparing PSA results with actual outcomes, the investigators then calculated the sensitivity and specificity of the PSA screening test for this unique population of men.

The specificity of the PSA test was 91 percent—that is, 91 percent of the men who were followed up and found free of prostate cancer tested negative. This percentage varied little by length of time from when the blood specimen was obtained to when the follow-up period ended. The sensitivity, on the other hand, was an overall 46 percent, but improved to 71 percent for the first through fifth years of follow-up. Sensitivity measures the proportion of true positive tests of all those who eventually developed the cancer; thus, 71 percent of those who developed the cancer within five years of the taking of the blood sample tested positive. This study increases our confidence in the PSA as a screening test for early detection of prostate cancer. The number of individuals who would have to undergo investigation because they were falsely labeled as "positive" is at an acceptably low level (specificity of 91 percent). The number of correctly labeled positive persons (the percentage of those who have the disease and are so indicated by the test) is also in an acceptable range (sensitivity of 71 percent). A baseline PSA level correctly identified 87 percent of all prostate cancers occurring within the first four years of follow-up. The test seems better at picking out the aggressive cancers: only 53 percent of the nonaggressive cancers were picked out.

This report suggests that the PSA test may be a valuable predictor of prostate cancer, but the problem of choosing the appropriate therapy remains. It is only after more randomized clinical trials are carried out to measure the efficacy of the various treatments that patients and doctors will have enough knowledge to rationally inform the choice of appropriate therapy for this common tumor.

The history of medicine contains many examples of new therapies or diagnostic procedures that were introduced without proper evaluation; then widely used until more careful investigation showed them to be ineffective or dangerous. The same kind of evaluation can prevent equally destructive mistakes in public health programs designed to prevent disease or detect it at an early and curable stage. The great cost of some of the newer technology has made its rigorous evaluation even more urgent. The epidemiologic methods for the task are there, if the public demand is sufficient.

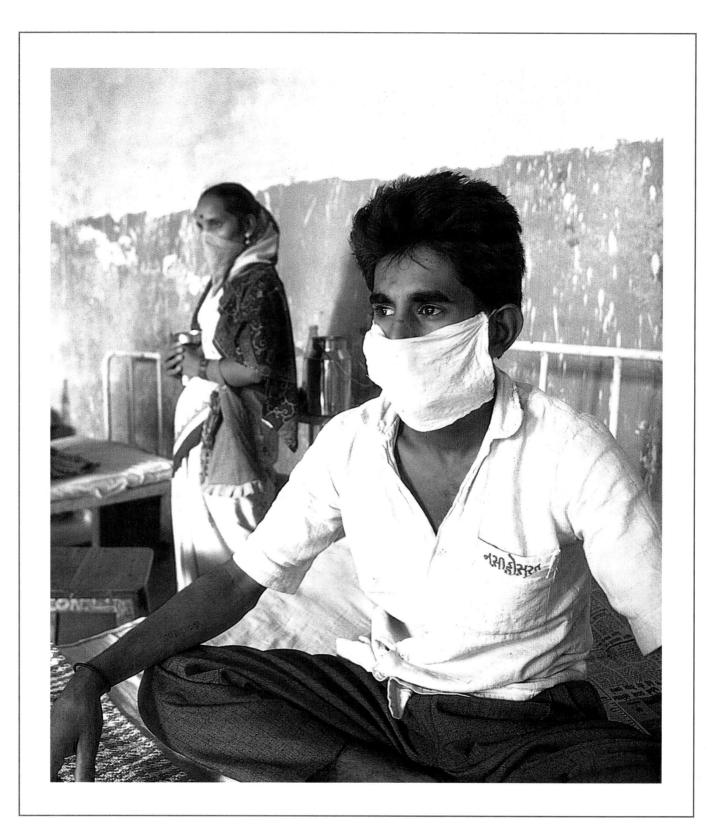

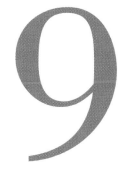

The Future of
Disease and
Epidemiology

A VICTIM of the bubonic plague, photographed in
the New Civil Hospital in Surat, wears a mask to
prevent the spread of infection. The recent outbreak
of the plague in this Indian city is a vivid
demonstration that infectious diseases have yet to be
conquered.

As epidemiology helps to illuminate the causes of an increasing number of health problems—including infectious diseases, cancer, cardiovascular disease, occupational disease, and others—we might wonder if, in the not far distant future, its major tasks may all be accomplished. Will disease be so well understood that there will no longer be reason to call upon the epidemiologic method? In fact, there is every reason to expect that the method will be as useful and fruitful in the future as it has been in the past, although the challenges to which it is applied may be quite different.

The infectious diseases, such as smallpox and plague, considered the major health threats of the last several centuries, are no longer a cause for concern in many parts of the world. In their place, though, new threats to our health are appearing. It is probable that the future will see chronic diseases (such as Alzheimer's disease), the health problems attendant upon population growth, and the violence and stress caused by the breakdown of society emerge as major health hazards. Nor have we seen the last of infectious diseases. Because of circumstances peculiar to the modern world, new infectious diseases are emerging at rates never before seen, and old ones are returning with renewed vigor.

Newly Emerging Infectious Diseases

IDEAS about ecology, evolution, and the environment all come together to help explain why the struggle to control infectious diseases appears to be never ending (except for some rare examples such as smallpox and poliomyelitis). Evolutionary theory predicts that pathogenic microbial organisms should become less lethal over many generations. The reason is conceptually simple: a parasite that kills its host will tend to die with the host, whereas a parasite that allows the host to live will continue to thrive and spread to other susceptible hosts. So, over time "natural selection" selects those variants of the parasite that are less lethal, and these less lethal types come to predominate. Tuberculosis may be an example: in the century immediately before the development of effective chemother-

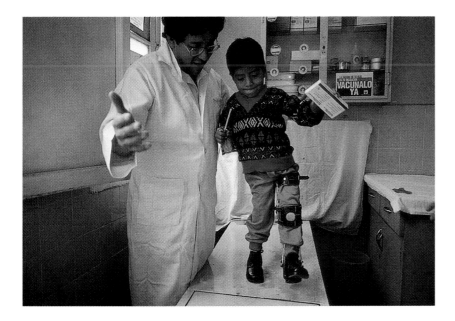

The last known child to be infected with polio in the western hemisphere takes a few steps at his doctor's request in Lima, Peru. If all goes as planned, vaccination campaigns will eradicate the disease throughout the world by the year 2000.

apy in 1950, the disease appears to have become "milder." Evolutionary forces also act on the host—in this case, the human host. Those individuals with the parasitic disease who survive are able to reproduce, and their genetic constitution is preserved along with whatever genetic factors endow resistance to the disease. Syphilis is another example of a disease that probably became less lethal over many centuries.

Therefore, over the long haul, the host and its parasites come into some sort of equilibrium: the parasites can get their "free lunch" without killing their host, and the host can survive the onslaught of the parasitic invasion. Indeed, over time the relationship between host and parasite may evolve in such a way that it becomes actually beneficial to the host. For example, the bacterial flora that inhabit the human gut provide the means to digest food in the colon. A newborn human infant has no gut microbial flora during the first hours after birth, and the gut must become colonized if the infant is to have satisfactory digestion.

When the equilibrium between host and parasite is disrupted, problems can ensue. A course of broad-spectrum antibiotics given to a woman to cure her bacterial sinusitis may also destroy the bacterial inhabitants normally present elsewhere in the body, allowing competitors to flourish. The result may be fungal overgrowth in the vagina, producing an annoying fungal vaginitis. Another rare complication of antibiotic treatment is a severe diarrhea attributed to *Clostridium difficile* in the lower gut.

In a similar fashion, but on a larger scale, when ecological equilibria are disturbed, diseases can emerge within a population. The crowding created as civil war impels mass migrations—such as occurred in Rwanda in 1994—increases the opportunities for infectious agents to be transmitted, and the accompanying stress and poor diet lower resistance to infectious diseases. Waterborne diseases resulting from the fecal contamination of drinking water are thus common in refugee camps and other places where large numbers of people are suddenly crowded together: cholera, typhoid fever, and shigellosis are examples of the diseases that may run rampant under these conditions.

New infections may be introduced into the human population when ecological relations are disrupted. In Chapter 1 we described how the great plague epidemic of the fourteenth century has been attributed by

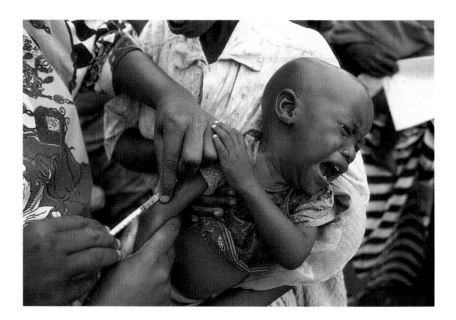

A child is vaccinated against measles in a Rwandan refugee camp in Tanzania. The crowded and unsanitary conditions of refugee camps encourage the spread of infectious disease.

some historians to a disturbance of the rat habitat in Asia. These historians suggest that the plague first spread to humans when crop failure and drought forced the rats into the homes of farmers and peasants. The domestication of animals many thousands of years ago brought pigs, cows, and fowl into close proximity with human habitats, and along with them came some of their parasites: trichinosis, leptospirosis, tuberculosis, and possibly even influenza.

AIDS, an apparently new disease in humans, may have come from a simian viral infection that was able to cross species and infect humans. The destruction of the habitat of lower primates, such as monkeys, along with the encroachment on their habitat by humans may have placed these animals into closer contact with our species and increased the chances that humans would pick up the viral infection.

Lyme disease, whose discovery was also described in Chapter 1, may have emerged as a new infection affecting human beings as a result of changing land use in the northeastern United States. Originally deforested during the Colonial era, that section of the country later became reforested and then subject to suburban residential housing development. Humans were living close together with deer, field mice, and their ticks and became the frequent target of tick bites. During its life cycle the vector tick, *I. dammini,* infests deer and mice; humans became an "accidental" host when their new land use patterns brought their homes close to the woods.

Another newly emergent infectious disease, Legionnaire's disease, may be thought of as a disease of advanced technology and its consequent disturbance of the natural ecology. The disease is caused by the bacterium, *Legionella pneumophila,* usually found in soil and water; apparently humans almost never contract it through contact with soil. Rather, the disease, a severe and sometimes fatal pneumonia, is contracted when the bacteria are aerosolized through air conditioning systems, as happened in Philadelphia during the Legionnaire's convention in 1976. The fans of the machines sweep the bacterium into the warm water surrounding air conditioning units (warm because of the heat exchange required in the cooling process). The warm water reservoir is a good growth medium for this bacterium, and the bacteria multiply. Large numbers are aerosolized and distributed through the air conditioning system, leading to human disease.

Recently, several alarming books *(The Hot Zone, The Coming Plague)*, television shows, and a popular, though fictional movie *(Outbreak)* have described some of the lethal and exotic viral diseases that have occasionally reached the United States, imported from the tropics of Africa and South America. Imported Lassa fever is the most commonly cited example of a newly emergent viral disease, dreaded because of its often fatal hemmorrhagic fever. In 1989 a case of Lassa fever was diagnosed in Chicago. Although the infected individual originally contracted the disease while on a visit to Nigeria, rapid air travel allowed him to arrive in the United States while still apparently healthy. After the infected man entered the country, over one hundred persons were known to have come into direct contact with him during his brief and fatal illness. Prophylactic ribavarin, an antiviral agent, was given to high-risk contacts, and fortunately no further cases occurred in the United States, but such infections may happen in the future given the ability to travel from one continent to another in only a few hours with modern jet aircraft.

There is a further ecological and evolutionary explanation for other emerging infections: drug-resistant tuberculosis, malaria, and gonorrhea, for example. Drugs that are initially effective may "lose" their efficacy over time, as the previously susceptible strains of pathogens become drug resistant. The resistant strains of the pathogens are either present initially or may arise as a result of random mutations, but no matter how they arose, the result is the same—the resistant strains survive and reproduce while the susceptible strains are killed. Eventually the resistant strains predominate, and the formerly effective drug no longer does the job. Currently, strains of tuberculosis, the gonococcus bacterium that causes gonorrhea, and the malaria trypanosome (a type of protozoan) are resistant to drugs that were effective only twenty years ago. Unfortunately, we are seeing the development of strains of the AIDS-producing HIV virus that are resistant to the drug AZT. Because the HIV mutates frequently, strains resistant to AZT eventually emerge in the infected individual and the drug loses its helpfulness—although only for that infected individual. In the other examples given, the resistant strains emerged in the population rather than in the course of a single individual's infection.

The widespread and often indiscriminant use of antibiotics is one cause of drug resistance among pathogens. Severe "head colds" are almost always caused by viruses not responsive to antibiotics, but some physicians used these drugs to treat colds in the early years of antibiotic therapy. Even now some patients demand them under the illusion that they cure or shorten a cold. However, these antibiotics may affect the bacteria that individuals normally harbor in the gut, skin, mouth, and throat. The population of any one strain is ordinarily contained by the competition for nutrients from other bacteria found in the same area of the body, but antibiotics can kill off susceptible strains of bacterial flora while antibiotic-resistant strains survive. Bacteria, normally kept in check, increase in number and may even act as pathogens. That is how the process of natural selection, so important in understanding evolution and population changes, operates in the human body when it is "fast-forwarded" by antibiotics.

Mosquitoes can acquire resistance to insecticides by the same mechanism of natural selection—an ability that has wrecked the campaign by the World Health Organization to control malaria in a good part of the tropics. The mosquito vector has "evolved" to become resistant to the commonly used pesticides, and the disease-producing trypanosome has similarly evolved in some parts of the world to become resistant to the drug chloroquine.

Population and Health

AFTER the great plague epidemic of the fourteenth century had wiped out as much as one-third of Europe's population, that population grew only very slowly as far as can be told from the poor records available. Although fertility was high, infant and childhood mortality were so great that a woman who bore nine or ten children might see only three or four reach adolescence. Most of these children who died young were the victims of infectious diseases encouraged by poor hygiene and sanitation that came from drinking contaminated water and living in proximity to domesticated animals. At that time, of course, there were no treatments or preventive measures against epidemic diseases such as diphtheria, small-pox, and pneumonia. Beginning about the eighteenth century, infant mortality began to drop for reasons that are not entirely clear, and the population of Europe began a remarkable rise that led to a great migration and the peopling of North and South America by Europeans. In the twentieth century, improved sanitation and the achievements of modern medicine have led to an even more dramatic rise in the populations of Asia, Africa, and the Middle East. The world population now stands at over six billion persons; China alone contains well over one billion and India nearly a billion. The population of some third world countries, such as Guatemala or Sierra Leone, doubles every 14 to 20 years. How has this unprecedented population increase affected human health? What are the challenges it creates for epidemiologists?

Overpopulation affects human health in many interconnected and sometimes subtle ways. It encourages disease through overcrowding, stress on the available food supply, and the accumulation of human and industrial wastes. Encroachment on the habitats of other species may lead to the emergence of new infectious diseases. The destruction of the ozone layer will increase the incidence of cancer. Global warming, if it occurs, is expected to disrupt the food supply. In addition, the increased poverty and disparities in wealth that may be one cause of conflict and war can lead to disease, famine, mass migrations, and violent death. While there are scientists who reject the scenario of a future dominated by the problems of uncontrolled human population growth, the majority of scientific opinion finds this view entirely congruent with what we know of the growth of other biological populations, be it rabbits in Australia or bacterial colonies in petri dishes: they will outgrow their food supply if population growth is unchecked.

If the food supply cannot keep pace with human population, famine must result. In this century alone the human "family" has experienced famine in China, India, Ethiopia, Somalia, the Sudan, and the former Soviet Union. Some economists argue that famine is usually found only in those countries that have no democratic governance; these countries are less likely to respond to pleas for food distribution when famine threatens and may even use the threat of famine as a tool of political repression, as the USSR did during the 1920s. Yet these arguments do not necessarily imply that famine would disappear if all countries adopted democratic political forms. Even democratic countries are likely to be overwhelmed when they can no longer maintain the narrow margin between sufficient food supply and shortage.

Along with the food supply, the supply of drinkable fresh water is threatened. The desertification of previously arable land, as is taking place in northern Africa, poses particular hazards to populations already residing in areas where water must be imported or is in extremely short supply.

Overcrowding and overpopulation tax the sanitary engineering infrastructure of even wealthy societies. One need only wander about Bombay or Cairo to see the dreadful consequences of urban overcrowding when combined with poverty. Sanitary facilities are completely absent in some areas of these large cities, and human excrement can be found in the streets as was commonplace in the Middle Ages. Dead bodies are seen lying in the streets of a city like Bombay, the deaths often a result of starvation.

Other effects of overpopulation are less direct. Since a growing human population will require increased energy, population growth will bring with it the increased use of fossil fuels or nuclear energy. The burning of fossil fuels produces air pollution and contributes to the destruction of the ozone layer. Nuclear energy poses the unique and presently unsolved problem of waste disposal. Pollution, ozone destruction, and waste are likely to be major health threats in the coming years.

Epidemiologists are already being called upon to investigate the poorly understood health consequences of air pollution from the burning of oil, coal, and gasoline. In future years they will also find their attention occupied with the possibly subtle effects of small doses of radioactivity. The United States has already experienced documented leakage of radioactive waste into the Columbia River system from the Hanford Atomic Bomb facility in Washington state. Since some of the wastes resulting from nuclear energy plants will remain radioactive for centuries, and no risk-free method of disposal is available, exposure to radiation is likely to remain a danger for a long time.

The Health Hazards of Societal Stress

THE complex relationship between the health of society and the health of the individuals who live in society is intuitively obvious but frequently forgotten. There is a dual responsibility for health: the *individual* is responsible for his or her habits and behavior, and *society* is responsible for the organization of health care, sanitation, automobile traffic, vaccination programs, and other community functions that can affect health. A society that has poorly organized and inequitably distributed health services, sanitation, housing, or food puts its members at greater risk of becoming ill and receiving inadequate care. For example, if government budgets are cut so that programs to help impoverished children receive their necessary vaccinations falter, the result will be the recurrence of epidemics of diseases, such as diphtheria, that are usually under control. While one can urge parents to take individual responsibility for arranging these vaccinations, barriers such as cost, access, convenience, illiteracy, and fear may prevent them. A well-organized public health system would provide a reminder of the need for vaccination, the vaccine when necessary, convenient vaccination stations, and so on.

How the dissolution of an effective public health infrastructure can lead to the emergence of a formerly controlled disease is illustrated by events in the former Soviet Union. The newly independent states created from the former Soviet Union after 1989 lacked administrative structures to continue the previously centrally administered public health activities. Vaccination of children became haphazard, and systems to measure vaccination rates were not operative. The level of childhood vaccination fell during this period of political upheaval and ethnic strife, and epidemics of diphtheria appeared. The disease, which in 1989 had afflicted 839 persons in the newly independent states, struck 47,802 persons in 1994, causing 1,746 deaths that year alone. Outbreaks of diphtheria have spread to adjacent areas, creating an international public health emergency requiring the intervention of the World Health Organization. Rapid travel and migration patterns now put all peoples at risk when public health measures fail in one part of the world.

Breakdowns in civil society can also contribute to trauma caused by violence, reckless driving, and sexually transmitted diseases. The application of epidemiological methods to the study of murder, suicide, and other human behaviors is one of the field's most interesting developments. In the United States, homicide is the leading cause of death in young African-American males, and most of these deaths are a result of handgun injury. A population of about 260 million persons has circulating in it an estimated 60 million handguns whose manufacture, distribution, and licensing is little regulated. There are few societies in the history of humankind where small weapons of such lethality were so readily available, and surely the easy access to handguns has contributed to at least some of the astounding homicide rates recorded in the United States in recent decades. The epidemiology of homicide is remarkable in that the majority of these murders occur on weekends, near bars or in homes, and among people who have been drinking heavily. Most often, the victim and the assailant are acquainted with each other at the time of the murder. Only a small minority of homicides are committed during the execution of another crime such as theft. While the individual psychology and infant development of the murderer may be of interest, the most successful public health response is one that tries to intervene by limiting the availability of weapons, places for assaults to occur, and public alcohol consumption and possibly by changing attitudes about how to respond to the aggressive behavior of others.

The public health approach to seemingly intractable health problems, such as homicide and suicide, is well illustrated by the United Kingdom's decision to try to cut its suicide rate through the simple addition of a noxious chemical to home heating/cooking gas. Suicide by asphyxiation (head in the oven with the unlit gas on) was the most popular method of suicide in the United Kingdom about three decades ago. The addition of the noxious chemical made this method of suicide very difficult: the individual trying it began to cough and feel sick before he or she had time to become asphyxiated. Surprisingly, after treatment of the gas had been instituted, the suicide rate declined even as people switched to other methods. That decline remained more or less permanent over the ensuing years, even though individual psychology probably was unchanged. Some argue that if the United States drastically reduced the availability of handguns, the homicide rate would fall even if the number of personal assaults remained stable: assault would perforce more often be carried out using a less lethal weapon.

The Molecular Biology Revolution and the Future of Epidemiology

THE revolution in molecular biology that began over three decades ago with the discovery of the structure of DNA has profoundly affected the field of epidemiology. New technology and methods are available to help answer the usual questions about disease patterns: Who develops a disease and why?

New techniques allow the epidemiologist to search for hidden viruses in the population under study. Such techniques have, for example, identified the human papilloma virus (HPV) as the most probable cause of cancer of the female cervix. Carriers of the HIV virus who do not yet show symptoms of the AIDS disease can be identified using the modern ELISA test for antibodies to the virus. The test has made the course of the epidemic far easier to track.

Modern immunological and genetic techniques have revolutionized the making of vaccines to control infectious diseases. Specific antigens of the pathogen (parts of the surface recognized by antibodies) can be isolated and used to prepare effective but safe vaccines. The hepatitis B vaccine is an example of a so-called genetically engineered vaccine that, although still quite expensive, is proving effective. Indeed, it may be considered an anticancer vaccine in that chronic hepatitis B infection is now known to be the most important cause of liver cancer in the developing world.

We can expect to see even greater application of modern molecular biological techniques to epidemiological problems in the future. Biological surrogate markers for exposure to harmful substances are being actively explored at this writing. Can some biological marker serve as an estimate of the exposure to a toxin, especially at the workplace? An example of such a marker can be seen in the chromosomes of persons occupationally exposed to the toxic gas ethylene oxide (EO). Each of us has 46 chromosomes in 23 pairs; sometimes during cell division the members of a pair exchange pieces of chromosome. More of these exchanges seem to have taken place in people exposed to ethylene oxide—that is, their chromosomes show the presence of larger amounts of "sister chromatid exchanges."

Ethylene oxide is used to sterilize many medical products because it can seep through packaging to the items in need of sterilization, such as a hypodermic syringe and needle. After the item, already in its sealed package, is placed in a sterilizer, the gas penetrates the packaging and disrupts the DNA of any microbes it comes in contact with, killing the microbes and producing a sterile package. Unfortunately, sterilizer operators run the risk of excessive exposure to this toxic gas. One of its early effects is to increase the number of sister chromatid exchanges seen in a certain type of white blood cell. Thus the increase in the number of exchanges can be considered a "surrogate" measure of EO exposure. Since the gas's rapid breakdown to harmless by-products makes the actual exposure to EO in the past almost impossible to measure, this surrogate measure may prove useful both in monitoring exposure and in characterizing the EO exposure of individuals participating in epidemiological studies. Proxy biological markers are now being developed to measure past exposure to very low levels of lead and mercury. These markers will be used in cohort and case-control studies of the possible toxic effects of low levels of exposure to these metals.

Health and Disease in the Next Millennium

FROM the time humankind began to record its history until the very recent past, infectious diseases were its greatest enemy and the main cause of mortality. Only within perhaps the last one hundred years did this pattern shift in the developed world. No longer was the expected pattern one of early death and high infant mortality, both from infection; rather, the pattern shifted to one of increased life expectancy and low infant mortality brought about by the successful control of much infectious disease through improvements in sanitation and hygiene, better housing, effective vaccines and antibiotics, and probably improved nutrition. Very quickly, the now longer-lived populations began to experience different patterns of disease. The so-called chronic or degenerative diseases began to dominate mortality. Heart disease, cancer, stroke, diabetes, hypertension, and death from accident and even suicide and homicide became prominent. Coronary heart disease, many cancers, and much diabetes can be considered diseases of improper nutrition (or "overnutrition") and the use of cigarettes. In some ways this is good news because it suggests that these diseases can be controlled by making life style changes. In fact, there is now evidence that coronary heart disease is declining. Since cigarette smoking is also falling in the United States, we should soon see a drop in the lung cancer death rate as well.

Meanwhile, sanitary conditions are still primitive in much of the developing world, and the mortality pattern is much like that of the developed world one hundred years ago, although many countries are beginning to control infectious disease and shift to a pattern of increasing chronic disease. The AIDS epidemic may interrupt that shift in much of Africa, however, as it has spread widely through that continent with devastating effect, wrecking the economies of a few countries already. The promotion of cigarettes in the developing world—with the profits funneling back to the West—raises the possibility that the people of the third world will repeat some of the West's mistakes.

The disease patterns of the future will be so dependent on the world political situation that one must project two scenarios: one for a relatively peaceful world of restrained population growth; the other for a world of constant strife and armed conflict as well as soaring population growth.

In a world where most nations can resolve conflicts peacefully and limit population growth, we can envision that more comprehensive and effective vaccination programs will bring infectious diseases under even firmer control. Cigarette smoking may begin to disappear and cancer rates drop as nations implement more successful campaigns to discourage the habit. Better nutrition should reduce the toll from heart disease, diabetes, and hypertension. Emergent new infectious diseases are a "wild card" and likely to increase as humans invade previously untouched habitats, where they will encounter viruses with which they have previously avoided contact. The diseases that follow in the wake of war and the mass migrations precipitated by political upheaval can be avoided in this probably utopian scenario.

The other scenario spells disaster, and there will be little medical science can do to alleviate the suffering in the long run. Weapons of almost unbelievable destructive power can now annihilate entire populations. Famine and epidemic disease will be the fate of many of those still alive in the wake of a nuclear war or even a conventional war as widespread as was World War II. Famine caused by overpopulation, global warming, and destruction of the biosphere will eventually devastate vast areas if population growth is not placed under intelligent control through some means of international cooperation.

A more probable scenario for the next millennium will be something in between these two extreme visions of the future. The population will grow gradually, perhaps declining in some areas where the scarcity of food sets off famine; frequent but not international war will create the conditions for starvation and disease within contained areas. World government and effective international cooperation are possible although, recent events suggest, unlikely.

No matter what the future may hold, epidemiology will have much to contribute. Epidemiologists will track the cause and origin of both new and older diseases, evaluate therapies and public health programs, investigate and solve outbreaks of disease, and record the history of the rise and fall of disease in populations. And epidemiologists will serve to remind both health professionals and politicians of the primary mission of medical science: better health for all peoples.

Further Readings

Buck, Carol, Alvaro Liopis, Enrique Najera, and Milton Terris, comps. *The Challenge of Epidemiology: Issues and Selected Readings.* Scientific Publication N. 505. Washington, D.C.: Pan American Health Organization.

Bulpitt, C. J., ed. *Epidemiology of Hypertension.* Vol. 6. Handbook of Hypertension. Amsterdam: Elsevier Science Publishers, 1985.

Ciba Foundation. *The Value of Preventive Medicine.* Ciba Foundation Symposium 110. London: Pitman, 1985.

Eyler, John M. *Victorian Social Medicine: The Ideas and Methods of William Farr.* Baltimore: Johns Hopkins University Press, 1979.

Higgins, Millicent W., and Russell V. Luepker, ed. *Trends in Coronary Heart Disease Mortality: The Influence of Medical Care.* New York: Oxford University Press, 1988.

Holtzman, Neil A. *Proceed with Caution: Predicting Genetic Risks in the Recombinant DNA Era.* The Johns Hopkins Series in Contemporary

Medicine and Public Health. Baltimore: Johns Hopkins University Press, 1989.

Marmot, Michael, and Paul Elliott, ed. *Coronary Heart Disease Epidemiology: From Aetiology to Public Health.* Oxford Medical Publications. Oxford: Oxford University Press, 1992.

Maxcy, Kenneth F., M.D., ed. *Papers of Wade Hampton Frost, M.D.* New York: Oxford University Press, 1941.

McCarthy, Mark. *Epidemiology and Policies for Health Planning.* London: King Edward's Hospital Fund for London.

Morrison, Alan S. *Screening in Chronic Disease,* 2d ed. Vol. 19. Monographs in Epidemiology and Biostatistics, ed. Jennifer L. Kelsey, Michael G. Marmot, Paul D. Stolley, and Martin P. Vessey. New York: Oxford University Press, 1992.

Needleman, Herbert L., ed. *Low Level Lead Exposure: The Clinical Implications of Current Research.* New York: Raven Press, 1980.

Rosner, David, and Gerald Markowitz. *Deadly Dust.* Princeton, New Jersey: Princeton University Press, 1991.

Rosner, David, and Gerald Markowitz, ed. *Dying for Work: Workers' Safety and Health in Twentieth-Century America.* Interdisciplinary Studies in History. Bloomington, Indiana: Indiana University Press, 1987.

The Science of AIDS. Readings from Scientific American Magazine. New York: W. H. Freeman, 1990.

Selikoff, Irving J., and Douglas H. K. Lee. *Asbestos and Disease.* Environmental Sciences: An Interdisciplinary Monograph Series, ed. Douglas H. K. Lee, E. Wendell Hewson, and Daniel Okun. New York: Academic Press, 1978.

Snow, John, M.D. *Snow on Cholera, Being a Reprint of Two Papers.* New York: Hafner Publishing Company, 1965.

Stolley, Paul D., and Tamar Lasky. "Johannes Fibiger and his Nobel Prize for the hypothesis that a worm causes stomach cancer." *Annals of Internal Medicine 116* (9): 765–769 (1992).

Terris, Milton, ed. *Goldberger on Pellagra.* Baton Rouge: Louisiana State University Press, 1964.

Vessey, M. P., and Muir Gray, eds. *Cancer: Risks and Prevention.* New York: Oxford University Press, 1985.

Wedeen, Richard P. *Poison in the Pot: The Legacy of Lead.* Carbondale, Illinois: Southern Illinois University Press, 1984.

White, Colin. "Research on smoking and lung cancer: A landmark in the history of chronic disease epidemiology." *Yale Journal of Biology and Medicine 63*: 29–46 (1990).

Sources of Illustrations

facing page 1
"The Plague in Rome," Jules Elie Delaunay, 1869, Musee d'Orsay, Paris. Erich Lessing/Art Resource

page 3
Colin McEvedy, "The bubonic plague," © *Scientific American, 258(2):* 122 (February 1988).

page 6
Explorer

page 7
Gail S. Habicht, Gregory Beck, and Jorge L. Benach, "Lyme disease," © *Scientific American, 257(1):* 81 (July 1987).

page 8
Russell C. Johnson, University of Minnesota

page 11
The Centers for Disease Control

page 12
Monty Roessel/Black Star

page 15
The Centers for Disease Control

page 16
CNRI/Science Photo Library/Custom Medical Stock

page 17
The Centers for Disease Control

page 19
David Levenson/Black Star

page 22
"Hiob," Otto Dix, 1946. V. G. Bildkunst, Bonn

pages 24 and 26
National Portrait Gallery, London

page 28
Wellcome Institute Library, London

page 30
National Portrait Gallery, London

page 33
National Library of Medicine

page 34
National Portrait Gallery, London

page 35
Wellcome Institute Library, London

page 39
Gary Cole/Biological Photo Service

page 40
Falk Library of Health Sciences, University of Pittsburgh

pages 41 and 42
Tom Pantages

pages 44 and 46
National Library of Medicine

page 47
Library of Congress

page 48
Albert G. Love, M.D., and Charles B. Davenport, *Defects Found in Drafted Men*, The War Department, 1920.

page 50
"Newsies at Skeeter's Branch, St. Louis, Missouri," Lewis Hine, 1910. Ford Motor Collection, Metropolitan Museum \

page 52
Sveriges Skorstensferjaremäsiksförbund

page 54
National Library of Medicine

page 55
Raymond Pearl, "Tobacco smoking and longevity," *Science, 87(2253):* 216–217 (1938).

page 57
Right side adapted from E. Cuyler Hammond, "The effects of smoking," © *Scientific American, 207(1):* 50 (July 1962).

page 58
Kobal Collection

page 60
Hygeia, 22: 422 (1944).

page 64
E. C. Hammond and D. Horn, "The relations between human smoking habits and disease rates: A follow-up study of 187,766 men," *Journal of the American Medical Association, 155:* 1316–1328 (1954).

pages 65 and 66
Staatsbibliothek Preussischer Kulturbesitz

page 67
University of the London School of Hygiene & Tropical Medicine

page 68
Data are from U.S. Dept. of Health and Human Services, *Reducing the Health Consequences of Smoking: 25 Years of Progress,* A report of the Surgeon General, 1989.

page 69
© American Heart Association, 1986.

page 70
K. E. Warner, "Cigarette advertising and media coverage," *New England Journal of Medicine, 312:* 384–388 (February 7, 1985).

page 71
Bruce Armstrong and Richard Doll, "Environmental factors and cancer incidence and mortality in different countries, with special reference to dietary practices," *International Journal of Cancer, 15:* 617–631 (1975).

page 72
The Wellcome Institute Library, London

page 73
Adrian Lee and Denise Lykos. Electronic manipulation by Jack Harris/Visual Logic

page 74
Right side adapted from Thomas Borén and Per Falk, "*Helicobacter pylori* binds to blood group antigens," *Scientific American Science and Medicine,* Sept./Oct. 1994.

page 75
Adapted from E. A. Stanbridge, "Identifying tumor suppressor genes in human colorectal cancer," *Science, 247:* 12–13 (1990).

page 78
From Jonathan D. Oliner, "The role of p53 in cancer development," *Scientific American Science and Medicine,* Sept./Oct. 1994, p. 17.

page 80
The Royal Collection © Her Majesty Queen Elizabeth II

page 83
The Francis A. Countway Library of Medicine

page 86
Stuart Franklin/Magnum

page 88
W. B. Kannel, P. Sorlie, W. P. Castelli, and D. L. McGee, "Blood pressure and survival after myocardial infarction: The Framingham Study," *American Journal of Cardiology, 45:* 326 (1980).

page 90
© American Heart Association, 1985.

page 93
Edimedia

page 98
Lipid Research Clinics Program, "The Lipid Research Clinics Coronary Prevention Trial results: I. Reduction in incidence of coronary heart disease," *Journal of the American Medical Association, 251(3):* 351–364 (1984).

page 100
Adapted from M. S. Brown and J. L. Goldstein, "Receptor-mediated endocytosis: insights from the lipoprotein receptor system," *Proceedings of the National Academy of Sciences USA, 76:* 3330–3337 (1979).

page 103
Adapted by H. W. Kohl II., K. E. Powell, N. F. Gordon, S. N. Blair, and R. S. Paffenbarger, Jr., "Physical activity, physical fitness, and sudden cardiac death," *Epidemiologic Reviews, 14:* 37–58 (1992), from David S. Siscovick, Noel S. Weiss, Robert H. Fletcher, and Tamar Lasky, "The incidence of primary cardiac arrest during vigorous exercise," *New England Journal of Medicine, 11:* 874–877 (1984).

page 105
World Health Organization

page 106
L. Goldman and E. F. Cook, "The decline in ischemic heart disease mortality rates: An analysis of the comparative effects of medical interventions and changes in lifestyle," *Annals of Internal Medicine, 101:* 825–836 (1984). In *Trends in Coronary Heart Disease Mortality: The influence of medical care,* ed. Millicent W. Higgins and Russell V. Luepker. New York: Oxford University Press, 1988.

page 108
Jeffery Wolin

page 111
Uffizi, Florence. Erich Lessing/Art Resource

page 113
Dr. Mohrmann, Dr. Raab, Occupational Disease Clinic, Bad
    Reichenhall

page 115
Archives and History Library, West Virginia Division of Culture
    and History

page 119
Personal communication from R. L. H. Murphy and B. G. Ferris
    to Irving Selikoff (1967), published in *Asbestos and Disease*,
    ed. Irving Selikoff and Douglas H. K. Lee. San Diego:
    Academic Press, 1978.

page 120
Dr. Mohrmann, Dr. Raab, Occupational Disease Clinic, Bad
    Reichenhall

page 121
Jeremy Burgess/Science Photo Library/Photo Researchers

page 122
Table IV from John M. Dement, Robert L. Harris, Michael J.
    Symons, and Carl M. Shy, "Exposures and mortality among
    chrysotile asbestos workers. Part I.: Exposure estimates,"
    American Journal of Industrial Medicine, 4: 399–419, 1983.

page 124
The Archives of the Mount Sinai Medical Center

page 126
National Library of Medicine

page 128
National Medical Slide Bank

page 129
Herbert L. Needleman, Charles Gunnoe, Alan Leviton, Robert
    Reed, Henry Peresie, Cornelius Maher, and Peter Barrett,

"Deficits in psychologic and classroom performance of
    children with elevated dentine lead levels," *The New England
    Journal of Medicine, 300(13):* 689–695 (1979). Figure 2,
    page 691.

page 131
Herbert L. Needleman, "What can the study of lead teach us
    about other toxicants?" *Environmental Health Perspectives,
    86:* 183–189 (1990).

page 132
Joseph L. Annest, "Trends in blood lead levels of the United States
    population," in *Lead versus Health: Sources and Effects of Low
    Level Lead Exposure*, ed. Michael Rutter and Robin Russel
    Jones. Chichester, G.B.: John Wiley & Sons, 1983.

page 133
Mark Asnin/SABA

page 134
Raymond Demers, "Overview of radon, lead and asbestos expo-
    sure," *American Family Physician*, Supplement, 51–56,
    November 1991.

page 138
"Hospital," Sesare Ciani. Gallera d'Arte Moderna, Florence/Art
    Resource

page 141
Hulton Deutsch

page 144
American Journal of Respiratory Diseases, 1972.

page 147
Neil Pearce, Richard Beasley, Julian Crane, Carl Burgess, Rodney
    Jacks, "End of the New Zealand asthma mortality epidemic,"
    The Lancet, 345: 41–43 (January 7, 1995).

page 148
Arthur L. Herbst M. D., "The Epidemology of Vaginal and Cervical
    Clear Cell Adenocarcinoma," Chapter 5 in *Developmental Ef-
    fects of Diethylstilbestrol (DES) in Pregnancy*. New York:
    Thieme-Stratton, 1981.

page 153
Swygert et al., Journal of the American Medical Association, 264 (20): 1698–1703 (1990).

page 155
March of Dimes Birth Defects Foundation

page 161
Paul D. Stolley, "Prevention of adverse effects related to drug therapy," in *Preventive and Community Medicine*, 2d ed., ed. Duncan W. Clark, M.D., and Brian MacMahon, M.D. Boston: Little, Brown & Co., 1981.

page 162
C. S. Perkins/Magnum

page 164
Sickles Photo-Reporting/Superstock

page 167
(left) American Cancer Society; (right) Erich Hartmann/Magnum

page 168
Institut de Virologie, Tours, France

page 169
D. MacTavish/Comstock

page 171
The Wellcome Centre Medical Photographic Library

page 177
Alan S. Morrison, *Screening in Chronic Disease*, New York: Oxford University Press, 1992.

page 178
S. Shapiro, L. Venet, P. Strax, et al., "Ten- to fourteen-year effect of screening of breast cancer mortality," *Journal of the National Cancer Institute*, 69: 349–355 (1982).

page 179
S. Shapiro, W. Venet, P. Strax, L. Venet, *Periodic Screening for Breast Cancer: The Health Insurance Plan Project and Its Sequelae*, 1963–1986, Baltimore: Johns Hopkins University Press, 1988.

page 181
Kathy Sloane/Photo Researchers

page 184
Peter Ginter/Bilderberg

page 188
"On the Clinic Stairs," Edward Steichen. Carousel Research/Eastman House

page 193
Lynn Johnson/Black Star

page 196
J. James/Science Photo Library/Photo Researchers

page 203
Marc B. Garnick, "The Dilemmas of Prostate Cancer," *Scientific American 270(4):* 76 (April 1994). Line art by Dimitri Schidlovsky. © 1994 Scientific American Inc., all rights reserved.

page 206
Swapan Parekh/Black Star

page 209
Karen Kasmauski/Matrix International

page 210
Steve Lehman/SABA

Index

Activity, heart disease and, 100–103
Adverse drug reactions, 143–149, 152–163
African Americans
    hysterectomy rates for, 199
    skin cancer in, 13, 70–71
AIDS, 211, 212–213
Alcohol, drowning and, 197–198
American Epidemiological Society, 44
American Journal of Epidemiology, 44
American Journal of Hygiene, 44
American Public Health Association, epidemi-
    ology section of, 44
American Red Cross, antidrowning campaign
    of, 197–198
Anemia, aplastic, chloramphenicol and, 160
Anitschkow, N.N., 90–91
Anthrax, 29
Antibiotics, 213
Antidrowning campaign, 197–198
Aplastic anemia, chloramphenicol and, 160
Asbestos, 112–125
    asbestosis and, 112–125
    dose-response relationship for, 116, 118,
        123, 124–125
    exposure to, assessment of, 118–124
    lung cancer and, 113, 124–125
    mesothelioma and, 113, 124–125

safe levels of, 118, 123–124
Asbestosis, 112–125
    exposure assessment for, 118–124
    history of, 112–118
Association, vs. causality, 65–67
Asthma mortality, isoproterenol and, 143–146
Atherosclerosis, cholesterol and, 90–100. *See
    also* Cholesterol

Baby powder
    coumadin contamination of, 159
    hexachlorophene contamination of,
        155–159
Baker, Dr., 126–127
Behavioral signs, of lead exposure, 127,
    129–131
Berlin, Jesse, 102
Biology, molecular, 218–219
Biological plausability, causality and, 136
Biopsy, prostate, 202
Birth defects, thalidomide and, 161–163
Black Death, 2–6
Blacks. *See* African Americans
Blinding, in clinical trials, 95, 192
Blood pressure. *See* Hypertension
Borrelia burgdorferi, 8

Bradford Hill, Sir Austin, 65–67
Bradford Hill criteria, 65–67
  in occupational epidemiology, 116, 136
Breast cancer
  genetic factors in, 76–79
  in nuns, 53
  radiation and, 143
  screening for. *See* Mammography
British cholera epidemic, 32–39
Broders, A.C., 54
Brown, Michael, 99, 100
Bubonic plague, 2–6
Buerger's disease, 13–14
Burgdorfer, Willy, 8
Byers, Randolph, 127

Cancer, 52–79
  breast
    genetic factors in, 76–79
    in nuns, 53
    radiation and, 143
    screening for. *See* Mammography
  causation of, 52–54
  cervical, screening for, 166
  diet and, 69–70
  genetic factors in, 75–79
  geographic distribution of, 12, 69–70, 73
  lip, pipe smoking and, 54–55
  lung. *See* Lung cancer
  occupational factors in, 11, 52–53
  prostate
    diagnosis of, 202
    screening for, 186–187, 201–205
    treatment of, 202–204
  radiation and, 141–143
  scrotal, in chimneysweeps, 52
  skin, 13, 70–71
  stomach, *Helicobacter pylori* and, 71–74
  uterine, estrogen and, 150–152
  vaginal, in DES daughters, 147–149
Cardiac disease. *See* Heart disease
Case-control studies, 19
  of asthma mortality, 136
  of breast cancer, 76–77
  of DES-related vaginal cancer, 147–148, 149
  of eosinophilia myalgia syndrome, 154
  limitations of, 63
  of lung cancer, 59–62
  nested, 204–205
  of occupational disease, 120
  odds ratio in, 61–62
  risk assessment in, 60–62
Case series, 144
Causality, 53–54
  vs. association, 65–67
  Bradford Hill criteria for, 65–67, 136
  in chronic disease, 65–67
  clinical trials and, 98
  dose-response relationship and, 67, 116
  duration of exposure and, 118, 124–125
  Henle-Koch postulates for, 65
  magnitude of effect and, 67
  in occupational/environmental epidemiology, 113–118, 135–136
  Selikoff's criteria for, 116, 124–125
Census data, 31–32
Cervical cancer, screening for, 166
Chalmers, Thomas, 194
Chapin, Charles V., 44
Childbirth (puerperal) fever, 140
Chimneysweeps, scrotal cancer in, 52
Chloramphenicol, aplastic anemia and, 160
Cholera epidemic, London, 32–39
Cholesterol
  heart disease and, 90–100
  in hypercholesterolemia, 99–100
  LDL, 96–97, 99–100
    regulation of, 99–100
  LDL receptor and, 99–100
  reduction of
    by diet, 91–94
    by drugs, 94–98
Cholestyramine, 94
Cigarette smoking. *See* Smoking
Clinical trials, randomized controlled, 94–98
  blinding in, 95, 192
  vs. cohort studies, 94
  for gastric freezing technique, 195–197
  for mammography, 177–178
  nested case-control study in, 204–205
  for portocaval shunts, 194–195

for selegiline, 192–193
for surgical procedures, 194–197
Cognitive impairment, from lead exposure,
    127, 129–131
Cohort studies, 19–20
    of DES-related vaginal cancer, 149
    Framingham Heart Study as, 86
    of lung cancer, 63–64
    of mammography, 171–172
    in occupational epidemiology, 120–124
    vs. randomized controlled clinical trials, 94
    reconstructed, 120–124
Colditz, Graham, 102
Congenital defects, thalidomide and, 161–163
Contingency (two-by-two) table, 61, 172–175
Controlled clinical trials. See Clinical trials,
    randomized controlled
Cooke, W.E., 112
Cornfield, Jerome, 61
Coronary heart disease. See Heart disease
Cost-benefit analysis
    for mammography, 179–180
    for prostatic specific antigen testing, 186
Coumadin, in baby powder, 159
Crimean War, mortality data analysis in,
    39–43
Cross-products, in odds ratio, 61–62
Cystic fibrosis, screening for, 182–185

Data collection
    census, 31
    questionnaires for, 16, 31–32
Death, during exercise, 102–103
Death statistics. See Mortality data analysis
Deer tick, Lyme disease and, 7, 8
Defoe, Daniel, 5
Dement, John, 121, 123
Depopulation, from plague, 4
DES-related vaginal cancer, 146–149
Devonshire colic, 126–127
Diagnosis. See Screening
Diagrams, 42
Diet
    cancer and, 69–70
    heart disease and, 91–94
    pellagra and, 46–49

Diethylstilbestrol (DES), 146–149
Diphtheria, 216–217
Disease(s). See also Epidemics and specific
    diseases
    causes of. See Causality
    classification of, 8–9
        Farr's system for, 32
    description of, 8–9, 24
    epidemiologic definition of, 10
    exposure and. See Exposure
    gender and, 11
    geographic distribution of, 8, 12
    germ theory of, 29–30
    iatrogenic, 141–163. See also Iatrogenic dis-
        ease
    incidence trends for, 56, 219–221
    natural history of, 9
    occupational. See Occupational epidemiol-
        ogy
    racial factors in, 13
    socioeconomic factors in, 13
Disease cluster, 9
Disease events, counting of, 25–27
Disease vector, 3
    identification of, 15–18
Doering, Carl, 55, 56
Doll, Sir Richard, 58–59, 60, 142
Dorn, Harold F., 69
Dose-response relationship, 67
    for asbestos, 118, 123, 124–125
    duration of exposure and, 118, 124–125
    for lead, 129–131, 134, 136
    in occupational/environmental epidemiol-
        ogy, 116, 136
Double blinding, 192
Doughty, Charles, 110
Drowning, prevention campaign for, 197–198
Drugs
    clinical trials for, 94–98, 192–193
    regulation of, 159–163
    side effects of, 143–149, 152–163
Dry bellyache, 126
Dry gripes, 126
Duodenal ulcers, gastric freezing technique
    for, clinical trial for, 195–197
Dust, lung disease and, 109–137

Ecology, 44
Economic factors. *See* Cost-benefit analysis
Education. *See* Public education
Elvehjem, C.A., 48
Emotional factors, in heart disease, 103–105
Employment. *See under occupation*
Environmental epidemiology. *See also* Occu-
    pational epidemiology
    causality in, 113–118, 135–136
    lead exposure and, 125–137. *See also* Lead
        exposure
Environmental hazards, 109–137
    asbestos as, 112–125
    exposure to, assessment of, 118–124
    lead as, 125–137
    political aspects of, 111–112
    safe levels of, 111–112, 123–124
Eosinophilia myalgia syndrome (EMS),
    153–154
Epidemics. *See also* Disease(s)
    causes of. *See* Causality
    characteristics of, 6, 10–14
    definition of, 6
    gender and, 11
    occupation and, 11
    spot-mapping of, 11–12, 156–157
    types of, 6
Epidemics (Hippocrates), 24
Epidemiology
    definition of, 9–10
    ecology in, 44
    in eighteenth century, 28–30
    environmental, 109–137. *See also* Environ-
        mental epidemiology
    field work in, 14–18
    focus in
        on behavioral changes, 69
        on disease prevention, 69
        on noninfectious diseases, 43–45,
            49
    future of, 207–221
    goals of, 10
    history of, 24–49
    of iatrogenic diseases, 139–163
    in nineteenth century, 30–43
    of noninfectious diseases, 43–45, 49

occupational, 109–137. *See also* Occupa-
    tional epidemiology
    professionalization of, 43–45
    public policy and, 39–43, 67
    scope of, 9–10, 43–45, 49
    in seventeenth century, 25–27
    uses of, 20–21
Estrogen, uterine cancer and, 150–152
Estrone, 152
Ethical issues, in clinical trials, 97–98
Ethnic background, 13–14
Ethylene oxide, 219
Exercise
    heart disease and, 100–103
    sudden death during, 102–103
Experimental hypothesis. *See* Hypothesis
Exposure
    definition of, 10
    duration of, 118, 124–125
    monitoring of, 119, 120
    occupational, 11
        assessment of, 118–124
        cancer and, 52–53
    safe levels for, 118, 123–124

False negative, 174
False positive, 170, 172, 173
Falsification, of hypothesis, 18–19
Family studies, 76–77
Farr, William, 30–32, 34, 38
    Florence Nightengale and, 39–43
Fat, dietary, heart disease and, 90–100
Feminine Forever, 150
Fibiger, Johannes, 53
Field work, 14–18
Fisher, R.A., 63
Fish tapeworm infection, 12–13
Fleas, plague and, 2–3
Food and Drug Act, 160
Framingham Heart Study, 86–90
Franklin, Benjamin, 126, 127
Freeman, Allen, 44
Friedman, Meyer, 105
Frost, Wade Hampton, 44–45

Gastric cancer, *Helicobacter pylori* and, 71–74
Gastric freezing technique, 195–197
Gender-related distribution, 11
General Register Office (London), 31–32, 38, 43
Genetic mutations
    hypercholesterolemia and, 99–100
    screening for. *See* Genetic screening
Genetics, of cancer, 75–79
Genetic screening, 180–185
    accuracy of, 181–182
    for cystic fibrosis, 182–185
    goal of, 181
    predictive value of, 181–182
    uses of, 185
Geographic mapping, 8, 11–12, 69–70, 156–157
    of cancer, 69–70
Germ theory of disease, 29–30
Goldberger, Joseph, 45–49
Goldstein, Joseph, 99, 100
Graham, Evart, 58, 59, 60
Graphs, 42
Graunt, John, 25, 27
Great Plague, 2–6

Haenszel, William, 69
Hamilton, Alice, 11
Hammond, E. Cuyler, 63–64
Harting, F.H., 52
Harvey, William, 82
Hawk's Nest Tunnel, 115
Hazardous materials. *See* Environmental hazards
Health care reform, Florence Nightingale and, 39–43
Health care system, evaluation of, 190–205
Health education. *See* Public education
Heart disease, 81–107
    Framingham Heart Study and, 86–90
    historical aspects of, 82–85
    mortality from, 85
        decline in, 105–107
    risk factors for, 86–105
        cholesterol as, 90–100. *See also* Cholesterol

        hypertension as, 89–90
        inactivity as, 100–103
        psychosocial, 103–105
Helicobacter pylori, stomach cancer and, 71–74
Henle, Jakob, 65
Henle-Koch postulates, 65
Hepatic cancer, occupational factors in, 11
Herbst, Arthur, 147
Heredity, 76–79. *See also under* Genetic cancer and
Hesse, W., 52
Hexachlorophene, in baby powder, 157
High-fat diet, heart disease and, 91–94
Hill, Sir Austin Bradford, 58–59, 60, 65–67
Hill, John, 54
Hill, W.H., 44
Hippocrates, 24, 140
HIP study, of mammography, 177–178
Hoffman, Frederick L., 114–115
Hormone replacement therapy, uterine cancer and, 150–152
Horn, Daniel, 63–64
Human immunodeficiency virus (HIV), 211, 212–213, 218
    screening for, 167
Hypercholesterolemia, 96–97
Hypertension
    heart disease and, 89–90
    lead exposure and, 135
    portal, shunts for, 194–195
Hypothesis
    definition of, 18
    falsification of, 18–19
    formation of, 19
Hysterectomy, evaluation of, 198–199

Iatrogenic disease, 141–163
    definition of, 141
    drug-induced, 143–149, 152–163
    hormone-induced, 150–152
    puerperal fever as, 140
    radiation-induced, 141–143
Ignatowski, A., 90–91
Incidence trends, 56

Intellectual impairment, from lead exposure, 127, 129–131
Ionizing radiation, cancer and, 141–143
Isoproterenol, asthma mortality and, 143–146
Ixodes dammini (deer tick), 8

Journal of the Plague Year (Defoe), 5

Kefauver amendment, of Food and Drug Act, 160
Kelsey, Florence, 162–163
Kessler, Irving, 69
Kidney disease, lead-induced, 135
King, Mary-Claire, 76–77
Kjerulff, Kristen, 199
Koch, Robert, 65

Laennec, René-Théophile-Hyacinthe, 82–83
LDL , 96
LDL-cholesterol, 96–97
   regulation of, 99–100
LDL receptor, 99–100
L-dopa, for Parkinson's disease, 191–192
Lead exposure, 125–137
   adverse effects of, 127, 128–131, 133–135
   history of, 126–129
   measurement of, 129–130
   occupational, 135
   safe levels for, 130–131, 132
   screening for, 127
   sources of, 128, 131–133
Lead nephropathy, 135
Legionnaire's disease, 10–11, 211–212
Lenz, W., 163
Leptospirosis, 15–18
Leukemia, radiation and, 141–143
Levodopa, for Parkinson's disease, 191–192
Life style changes, for disease prevention, 69
Lilienfeld, Abraham, 65, 69
Limb deformities, thalidomide and, 161–163
Lip cancer, pipe smoking and, 54–55
Lipid Research Clinics Coronary Primary Prevention Trial, 95

Lipoprotein, low-density. *See* Low-density lipoprotein
Lister, Joseph, 29–30
Liver cancer, occupational factors in, 11
Livingstone, Jean, 184
Lombard, Herbert, 55, 56
London cholera epdidemic, 32–39
London Epidemiological Society, 43–44
Lord, Elizabeth, 127
Louis, Pierre, 31
Low-density lipoprotein, 96
Low-density lipoprotein cholesterol, 96–97
   regulation of, 99–100
Low-density lipoprotein receptor, 99–100
Low-fat diet, for heart disease prevention, 92–94
L-Tryptophan, eosinophilia myalgia syndrome and, 153–154
Lung cancer, 52–79
   asbestos and, 113, 124–125
   increased incidence of, 56–58
   occupational factors in, 11, 13, 124–125
   smoking and, 54–69
      case-control studies of, 59–62
      causality criteria for, 65–67
      cohort studies of, 63–64
      early studies of, 54–58
      public education about, 68–69
      Surgeon General's report on, 67–68
Lung diseases, inhalational, 112
   asbestosis as, 112–125. *See also* Asbestosis
   silicosis as, 114–115
Lyme disease, 7–8, 211

Magnitude of effect, 67
Malignant melanoma, 13, 70–71
Malnutrition, pellagra and, 46–49
Mammography, 169–170
   cost-benefit analysis for, 179–180
   frequency of, 180
   patient selection for, 178–180
   risk-benefit assessment for, 143
   sensitivity of, 171–172
   specificity of, 171, 173, 174
   survival value of, 175–178

Mapping
    of cancer, 11–12, 69–70
    spot, 11–12, 156–157
Marshall, Barry J., 72
Martin-Bouyer, Gilbert, 158
Melanoma, 13, 70–71
Menopause, estrogen therapy in, uterine cancer and, 150–152
Mesothelioma, 113, 124–125
Meta-analysis, 102
Miners, silicosis in, 114–115
Miscarriage, diethylstilbestrol for, 147–149
Monitoring, of exposure levels, 119, 120
Montagu-Murray, H., 112
Mortality data analysis
    for British Army, 39–43
    in London cholera epidemic, 32–39
MPTP-induced Parkinsonism, 192
Muench's law, 195
Multiple regression techniques, 88–89
Multiple Risk Factor Intervention Trial, 91
Mutations
    cancer and, 76–79
    hypercholesterolemia and, 99–100
    screening for, 180–185. See also Genetic screening
        cystic fibrosis, 182–185

Nebulizers, isoproterenol, mortality from, 143–146
Needleman, Herbert, 128–129
Nephropathy, lead, 135
Nested case-control study, 204–205
Neurologic injury, lead exposure and, 127, 128–131
Nightingale, Florence, 32, 39–43, 190
Nutrition
    cancer and, 69–70
    heart disease and, 91–94
    pellagra and, 46–49

Observations on the Bills of Mortality (Graunt), 27
Occupational epidemiology, 11, 109–137. See also Environmental epidemiology
    asbestosis and, 112–125. See also Asbestosis

cancer and, 11, 52–53, 113, 124–125
case-control studies in, 120
causality in, 113–118, 135–136
dose-response relationship in, 116, 118, 123, 124–125, 136
exposure assessment in, 118–124
heart disease and, 104
history of, 110–112
lead poisoning and, 135
political factors in, 111–112
reconstructed cohort studies in, 120–124
silicosis and, 114–115
Odds ratio, calculation of, 61–62
On the Mode of the Transmission of Cholera (Snow), 33

Palmerston, Lord, 40
Pandemic, definition of, 6
Pap test, 166
Parkinson's disease, selegiline for, 191–193
Pasteur, Louis, 29
Pearce, Neil, 146
Pearl, Raymond, 55
Pellagra, 46–49
Peptic ulcers, gastric freezing technique for, 195–197
Personality factors, in heart disease, 105
Petty, Sir William, 25–27, 31
Phenylketonuria (PKU), screening for, 180–181
Phocomelia, thalidomide and, 161–163
Physical activity
    heart disease and, 100–103
    sudden death during, 102–103
Pipe smoking, lip cancer and, 54–55
Placebo, 95
Plague, 2–6
Plausability, biologic, vs. causality, 136
p53 mutations, 77–78
Pneumonic plague, 4
Polio, 9, 11–12
Polio vaccine, injury from, 154–155
Popper, Karl, 18
Population growth, 214–215
Population loss, from plague, 4

Portocaval shunts, clinical trials for, 194–195
Poskanzer, David, 147
Pott, Percival, 52
Predictive value, of screening, 174–175
Premarin, 152
Prenatal screening, 181–185
Prevention, behavioral changes and, 68–69
Prospective cohort studies. *See* Cohort studies
Prostate biopsy, 202
Prostate cancer
   diagnosis of, 202
   screening for, 186–187, 201–205
   treatment of, 202–204
Psychosocial risk factors, in heart disease,
     103–105
Public education
   about hypertension, 89–90
   about smoking and lung cancer, 68–69
   for disease prevention, 68–69
   for drowning prevention, 197–198
   evaluation of, 197–198
   for seat belt use, 198
Public policy
   epidemiology and, 67, 216–218
   statistics and, 39–43, 67
Puerperal fever, 140
Pulmonary diseases. *See* Lung diseases
Pulmonary fibrosis, asbestos and, 112, 118. *See
    also* Asbestosis

Questionnaires, 16, 31–32
Quetelet, Adolphe, 40

Race
   hysterectomy rates and, 199
   skin cancer and, 13, 70–71
   vs. socioeconomic status, 13
Radiation, cancer and, 141–143
Radical prostatectomy, 203–204
Ramazzini, Bernardino, 53, 110
Randomized controlled clinical trials. *See*
    Clinical trials, randomized controlled
Rats, plague and, 2–3
Reconstructed cohort study, 120–124
Rectal digital examination, for prostate cancer,
    201–202

Rehn, Ludwig, 52
Renal disease, lead-induced, 135
Risk assessment, 60–62
Risk factors
   for heart disease, 86–105
   for lung cancer. *See* Lung cancer, smoking
     and
Risk reduction, public education for, 69
Rosenman, Ray H., 105

Salk vaccine, injury from, 154–155
Sartwell, Phillip, 65
Scientific method, 18–21
Screening, 165–187
   accuracy of, evaluation of, 170–175
   for breast cancer. *See* Mammography
   cost-benefit analysis for, 186–187
   for cystic fibrosis, 182–185
   genetic, 180–185. *See also* Genetic screening
   history of, 167–168
   for human immunodeficiency virus, 167
   increasing use of, 168
   for infectious diseases, 166–167
   for lead poisoning, 127
   limitations of, 170–171
   for noninfectious diseases, 168–167
   predictive value of, 174–175
   prenatal, 181–185
   for prostate cancer, 186–187, 201–205
   results of
     false negative, 174
     false positive, 170, 172, 173
     true negative, 171, 173
     true positive, 171, 173
   sensitivity of, 171–172, 173
   socioeconomic factors in, 186–187
   specificity of, 171, 173, 174
   survival value of, 175–178
   for syphilis, 167
   treatment and, 175–178
   for tuberculosis, 166, 167
Scrotal cancer, in chimneysweeps, 52
Seleginine, for Parkinson's disease, 191–193
Selikoff, Irving, 116, 124
Selikoff's criteria, for causality, 116, 124–125

Semmelweis, Ignaz, 140
Sensitivity, of screening test, 171–172, 173
Shunts, portocaval, clinical trials for, 194–195
Silicosis, 114–115
Siscovick, David, 102
Skin cancer, 13, 70–71
Skolnick, Mark H., 77
Smoking
    heart disease and, 85
    lung cancer and, 54–69. *See also* Lung cancer
    prevention of, 68–69
    public education about, 68–69
    as risk factor, 68
Smoking and Health (U.S. Surgeon General), 67–68
Snow, John, 32–39, 60
Societal stress, 216–218
Socioeconmic status, 13
Socioeconomic effects, of epidemidcs, 6
Sömmerring, Samuel von, 54
Sonogram, of prostate, 201–202
Soot wart, 52
Specificity, of screening test, 171, 173, 174
Sphygmomanometer, 83
Spiroptera carcinoma, 53
Spot-mapping, 11–12, 156–157
Statistics
    development of, 28, 30–32
    graphic depiction of, 42
    in health care reform, 40–43
Steere, Allen, 8
Stethoscope, 83
Stomach cancer, *Helicobacter pylori* and, 71–74
Stonecutters
    lung disease in, 110, 114–115
Stratified analysis, 87
Stress, heart disease and, 104–105
Sudden death, during exercise, 102–103
Super, M., 183, 185
Surgeon General's Report on Smoking and Health, 67–68
Surgery
    evaluation of, 194–197, 198–201

for prostate cancer, 203–204
    racial factors in, 198–199
Swimming safety program, 197–198
Sydenham, Thomas, 24, 29
Sydenstricker, Edgar, 47
Syphilis, Wassermann test for, 167
Systemic lupus erythematosus, gender and, 11

Table, two-by-two, 61, 172–175
Talcum powder
    coumadin contamination of, 159
    hexachlorophene contamination of, 155–159
Tapeworm infection, 12–13
Thalidomide, 160–163
Tick, Lyme disease and, 7, 8
Tine test, 166, 167
Tonsillectomy, evaluation of, 199–201
Toxic shock syndrome, 19
L-Tryptophan, eosinophilia myalgia syndrome and, 153–154
Tsui, Lap-Chu, 182
Tuberculosis
    fluoroscopy in, breast cancer and, 143
    screening for, 166, 167
Two-by-two table, 61, 172–175
Type A personality, heart disease and, 105

Ulcers, gastric freezing technique for, 195–197
Ulfelder, Howard, 147
Ultrasound, of prostate, 201–202
Uterine cancer, estrogen and, 150–152

Vaccine, polio, injury from, 154–155
Vaginal cancer, diethylstilbestrol and, 147–149
Vaughn, Benjamin, 127
Vector, disease, 3
    identification of, 15–18
Victoria, Queen, 32, 40
Vital statistics, 30–32

Warfarin, in baby powder, 159
Warren, J. Robin, 72

Wassermann test, 167
Water-borne disease, 15–18, 39
  cholera as, 32–39
  lead poisoning as, 132
Wedeen, Richard P., 133–135
White, Josh, 115
Winslow, Charles-Edward Amory, 24
Work. *See under occupation*

Wynder, Ernst, 58, 59, 60

Xenopsylla cheopis (rat flea), 3
X-rays, cancer and, 141–143

Yersinia pestis, 2
Yerushalmy, Jacob, 65